Prithvi Raj · Hans Nolte · Michael Stanton-Hicks

Illustrated Manual of Regional Anesthesia

Conception, Realization, Consultation, Organization: Bureaux Bassler, Karlsruhe, FRG
Artist: Wolfgang Rost, Graphic-Design

Part 3: Transparencies 43–62

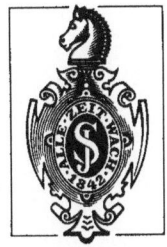

Springer-Verlag Berlin Heidelberg GmbH

ISBN 978-3-642-47803-1   ISBN 978-3-642-61391-3 (eBook)
DOI 10. 1007/978-3-642-61391-3

Dorsal approach for intercostal nerve block and thoracic paravertebral nerve block in prone position (see also Transparency 44, Sect. VII. B, and Transparency 45). ① Injection sites for dorsal intercostal nerve block. ⑪ Injection sites for thoracic paravertebral nerve block.
A – – – – A: Line intersecting spinous process of T3

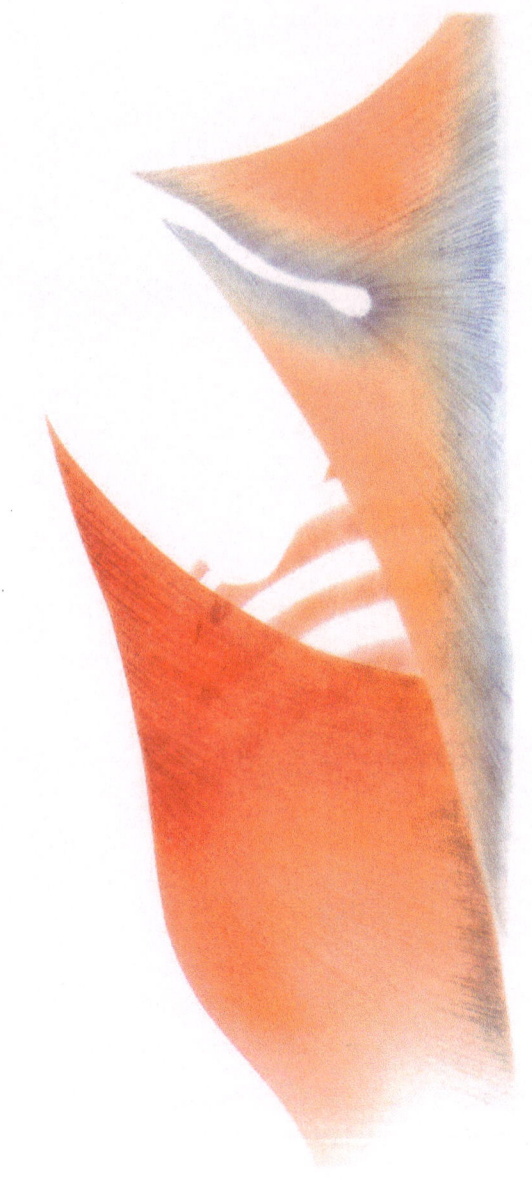

43.3

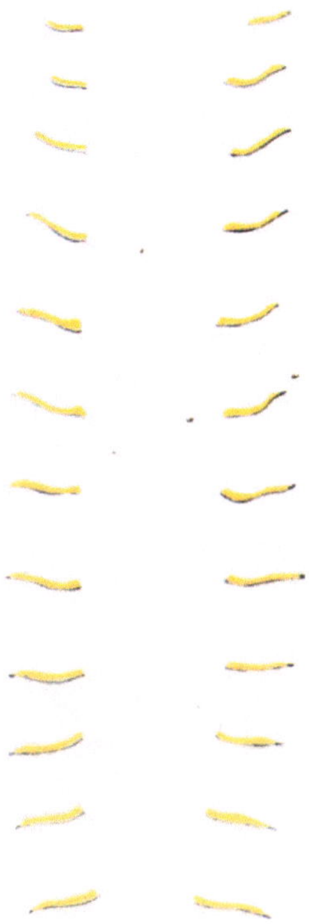

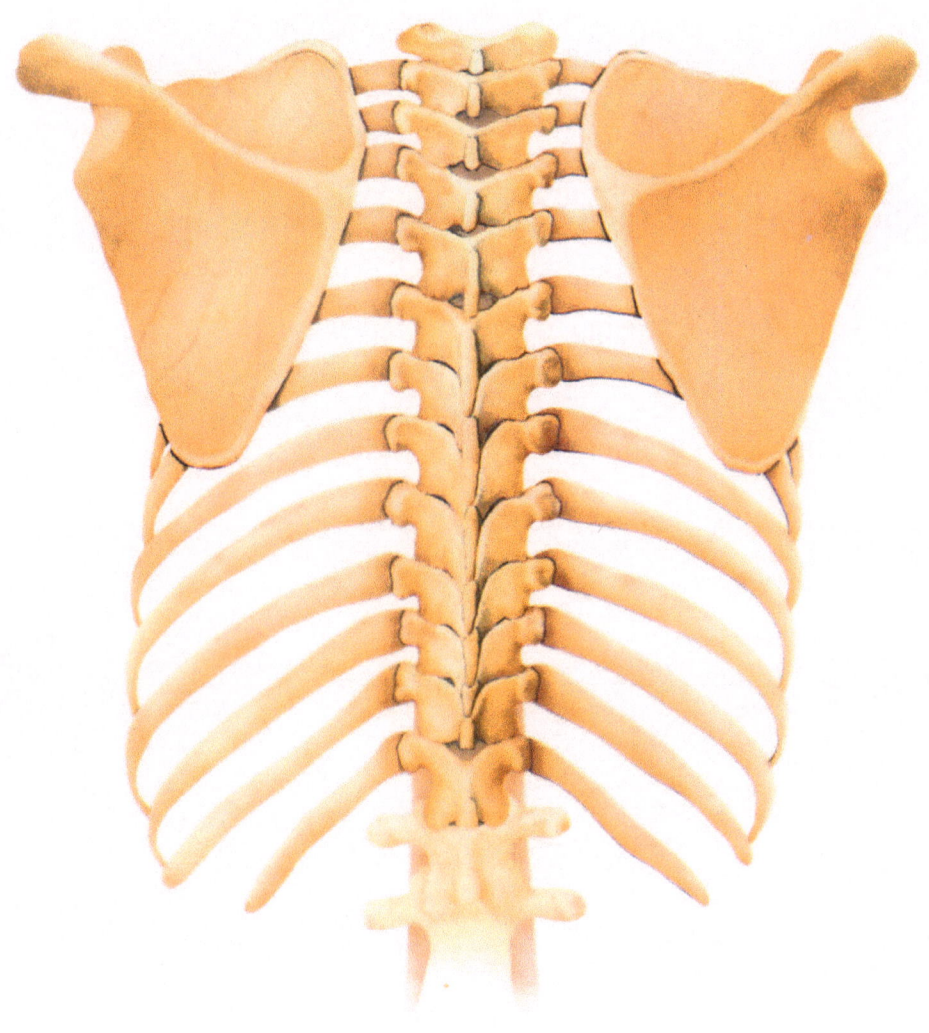

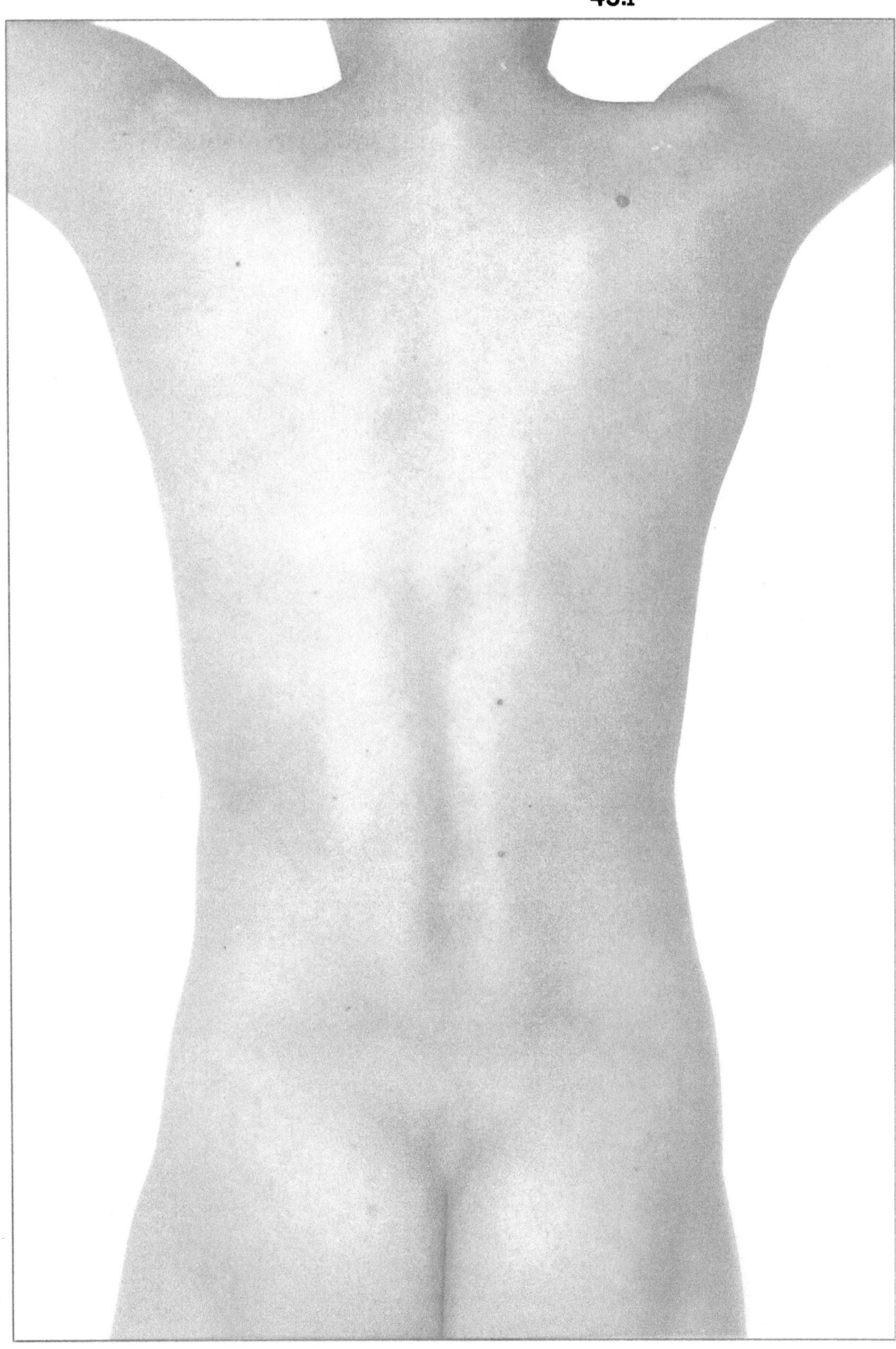

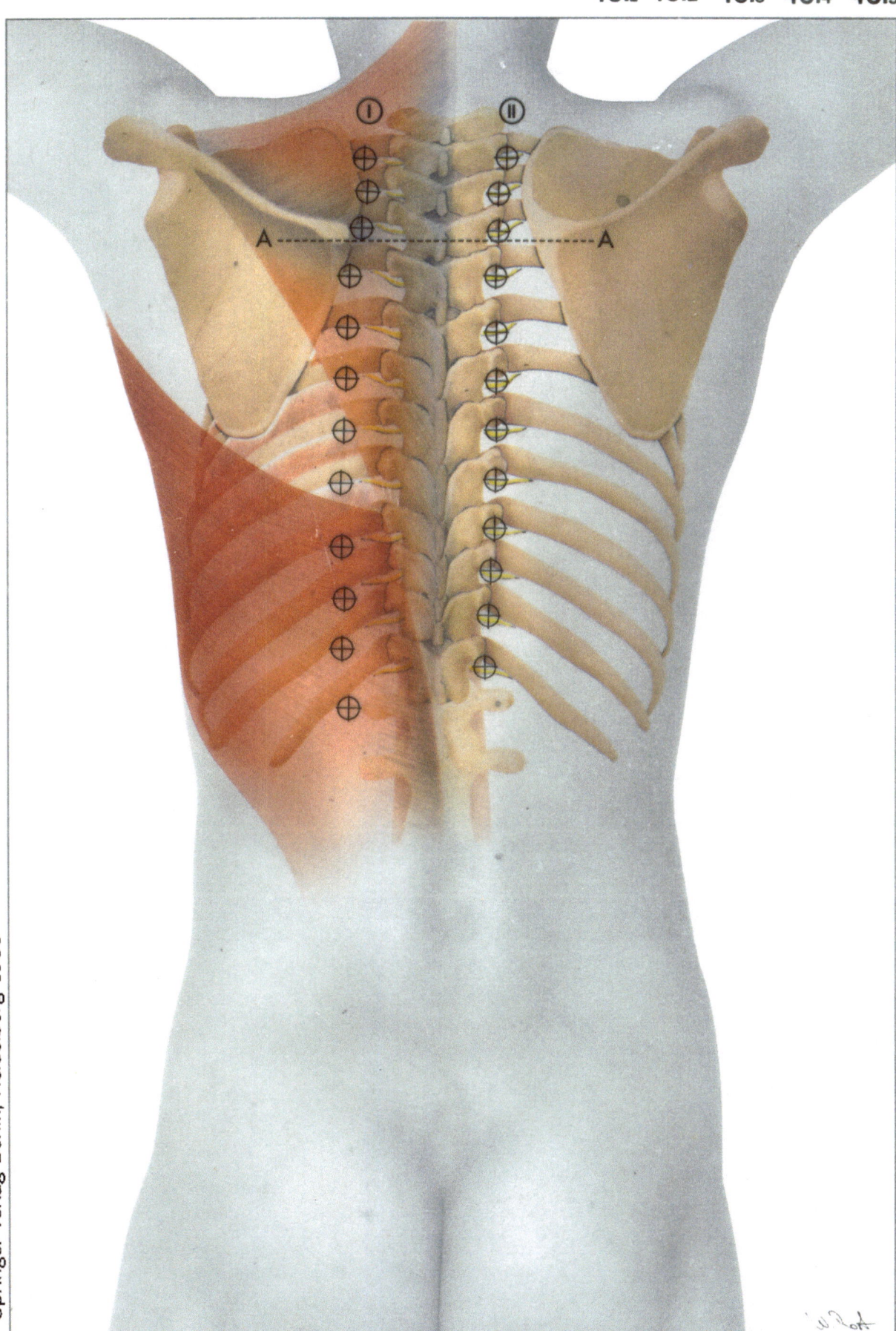

43

Dorsal approach for intercostal nerve block and thoracic paravertebral nerve block in prone position (see also Transparency 44, Sect. VII.B, and Transparency 45). ① Injection sites for dorsal intercostal nerve block. ② Injection sites for thoracic paravertebral nerve block.
A – – – – A: Line intersecting spinous process of T3

Anterolateral and posterolateral approaches for intercostal nerve block. ① Injection sites anterior to midaxillary line. ② Injection sites posterior to midaxillary line

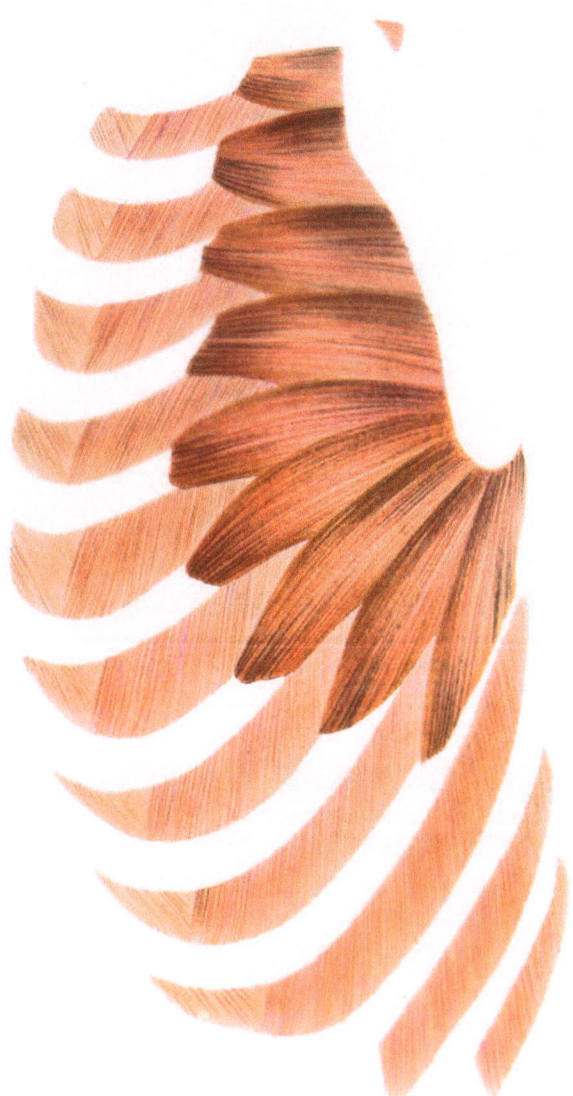

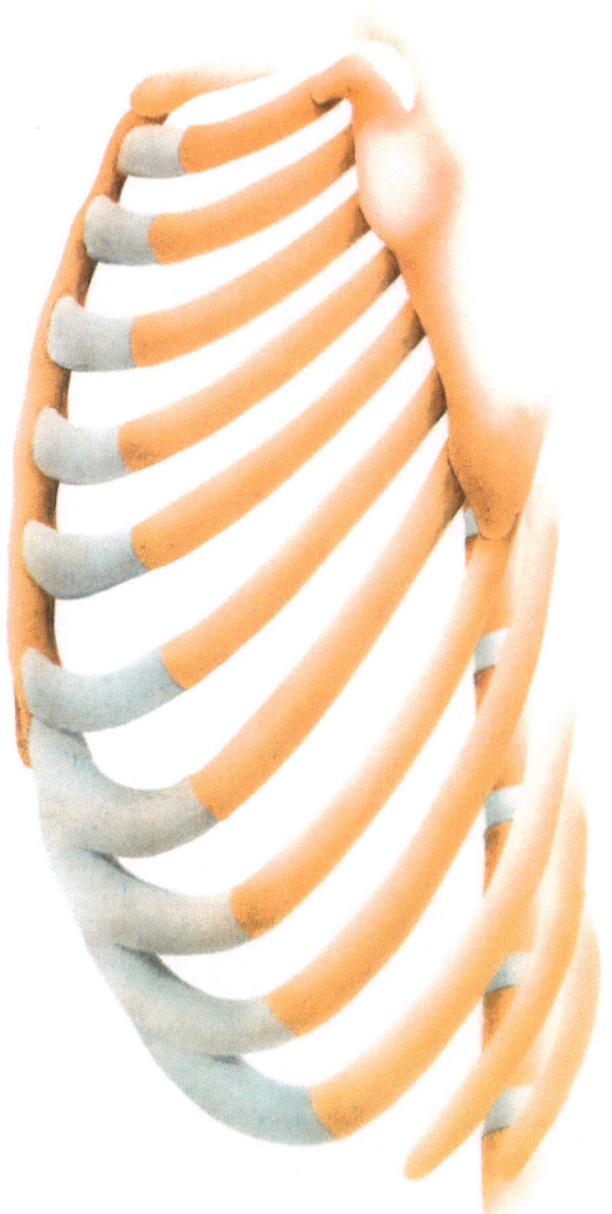

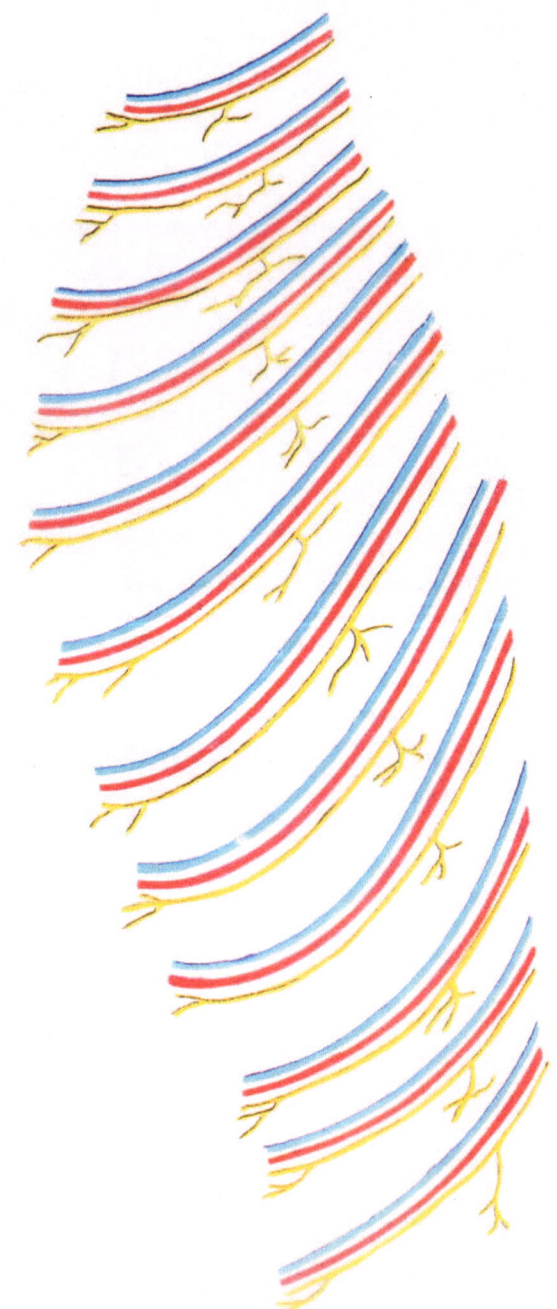

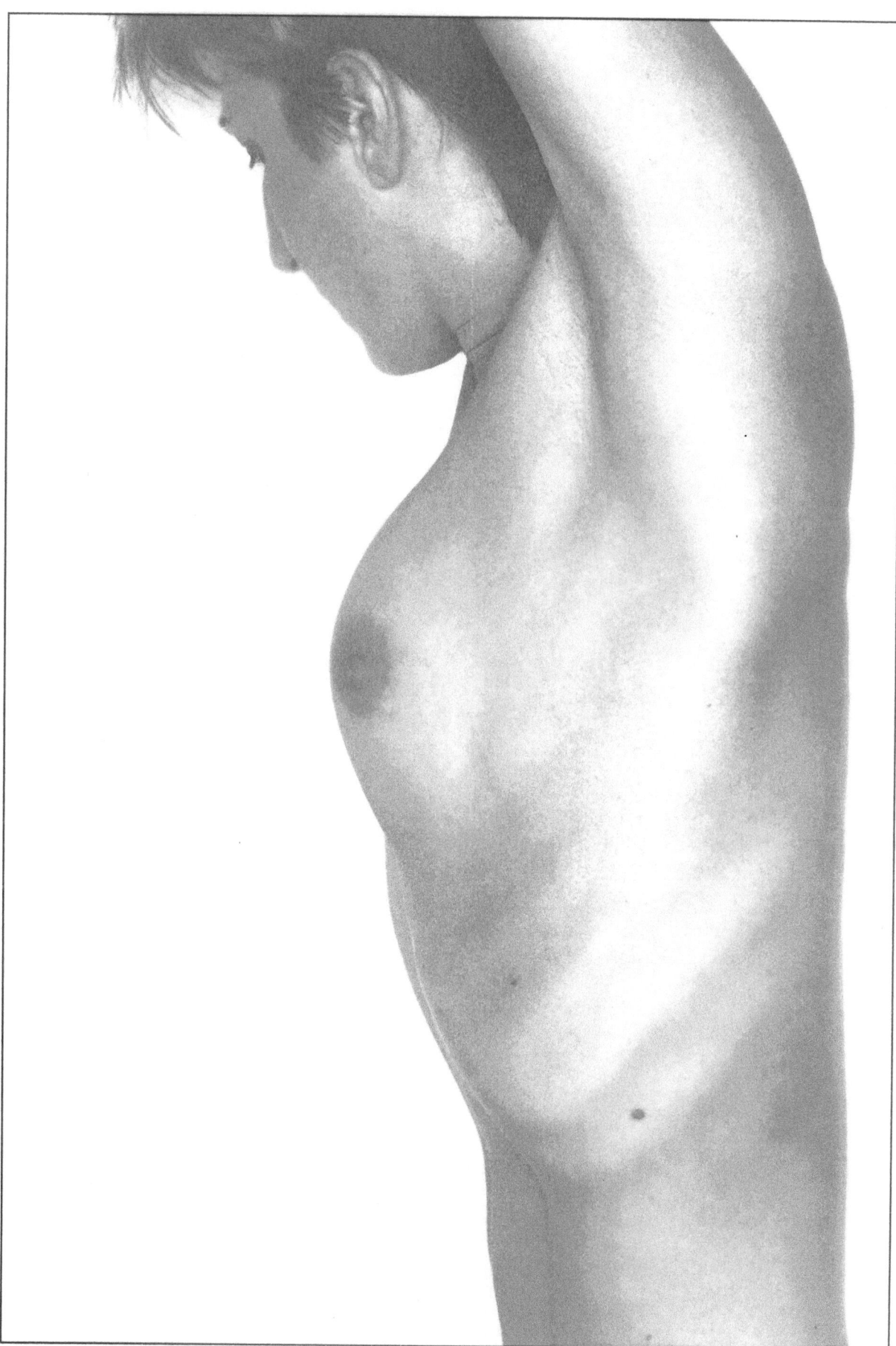

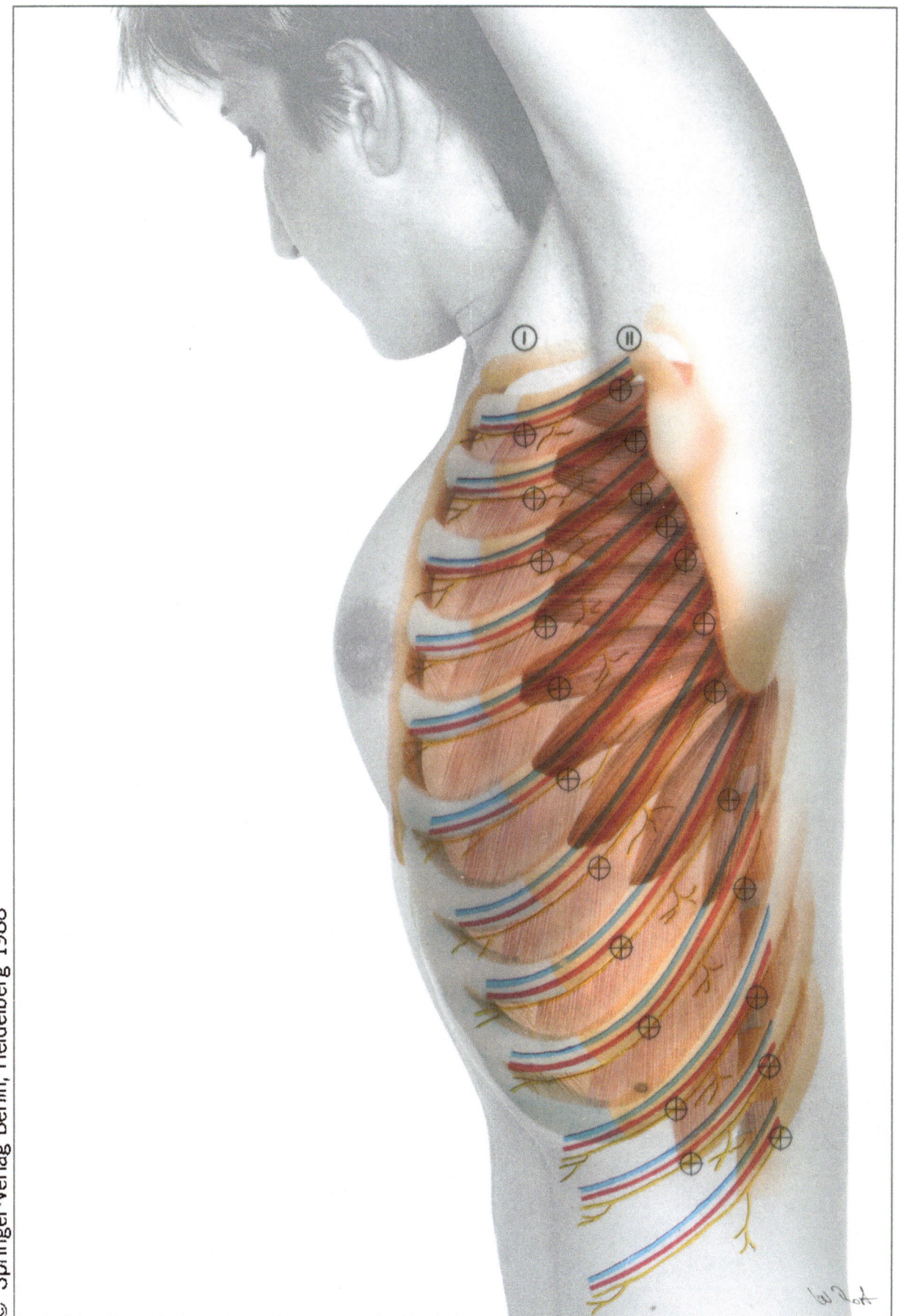

Anterolateral and posterolateral approaches for intercostal nerve block. ① Injection sites anterior to midaxillary line. ② Injection sites posterior to midaxillary line

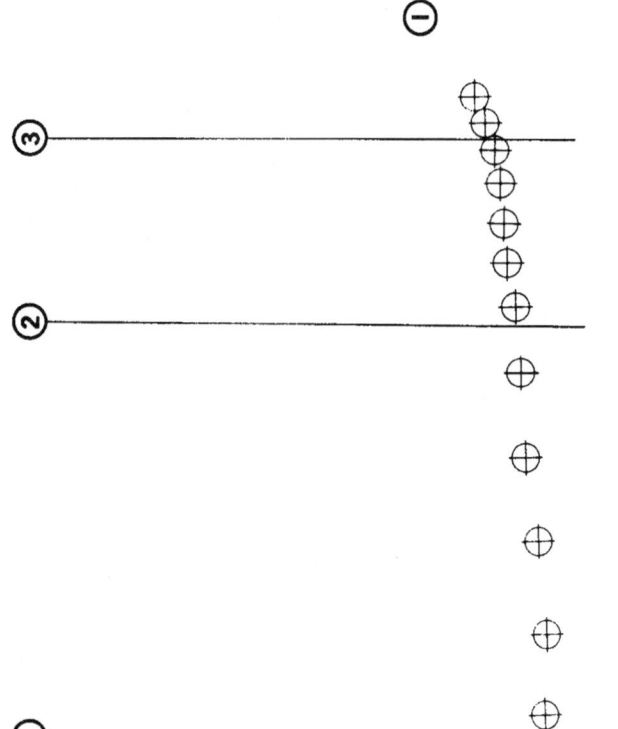

① Injection sites for thoracic paravertebral nerve block (with patient in lateral decubitus position). ① Spinous process of T12. ② T7–8 interspace. ③ Spinous process of T3

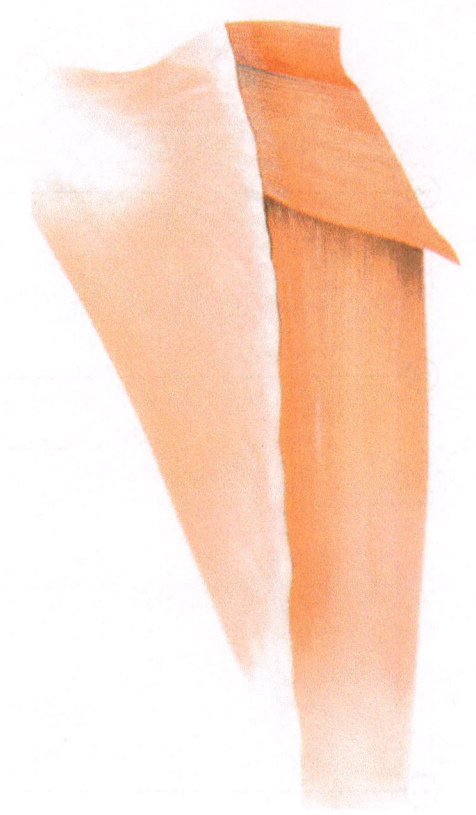

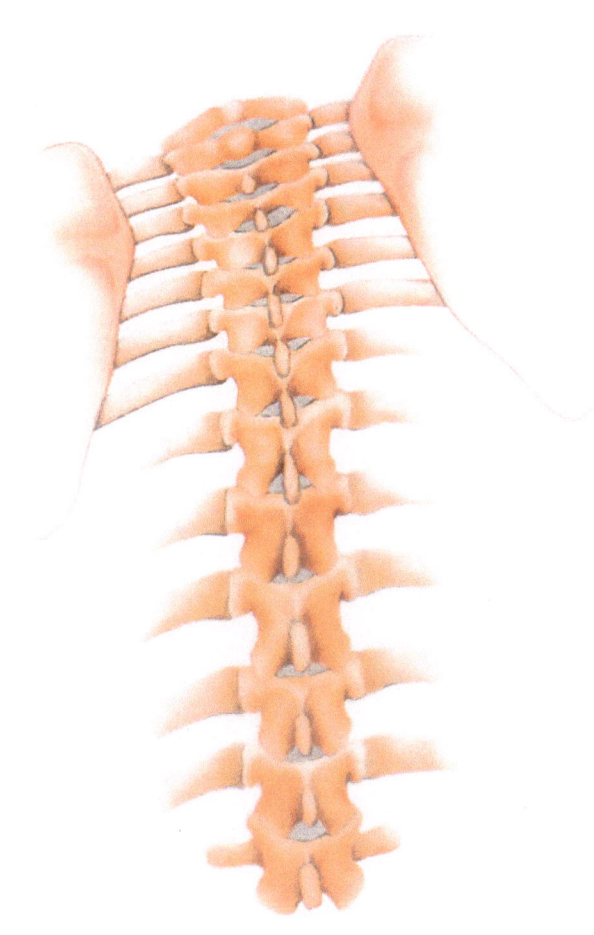

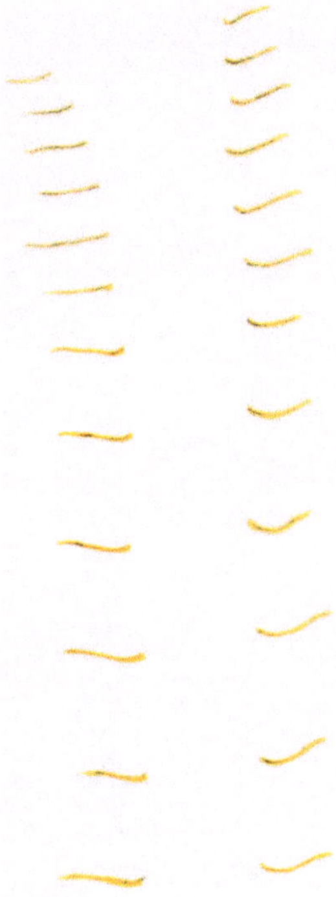

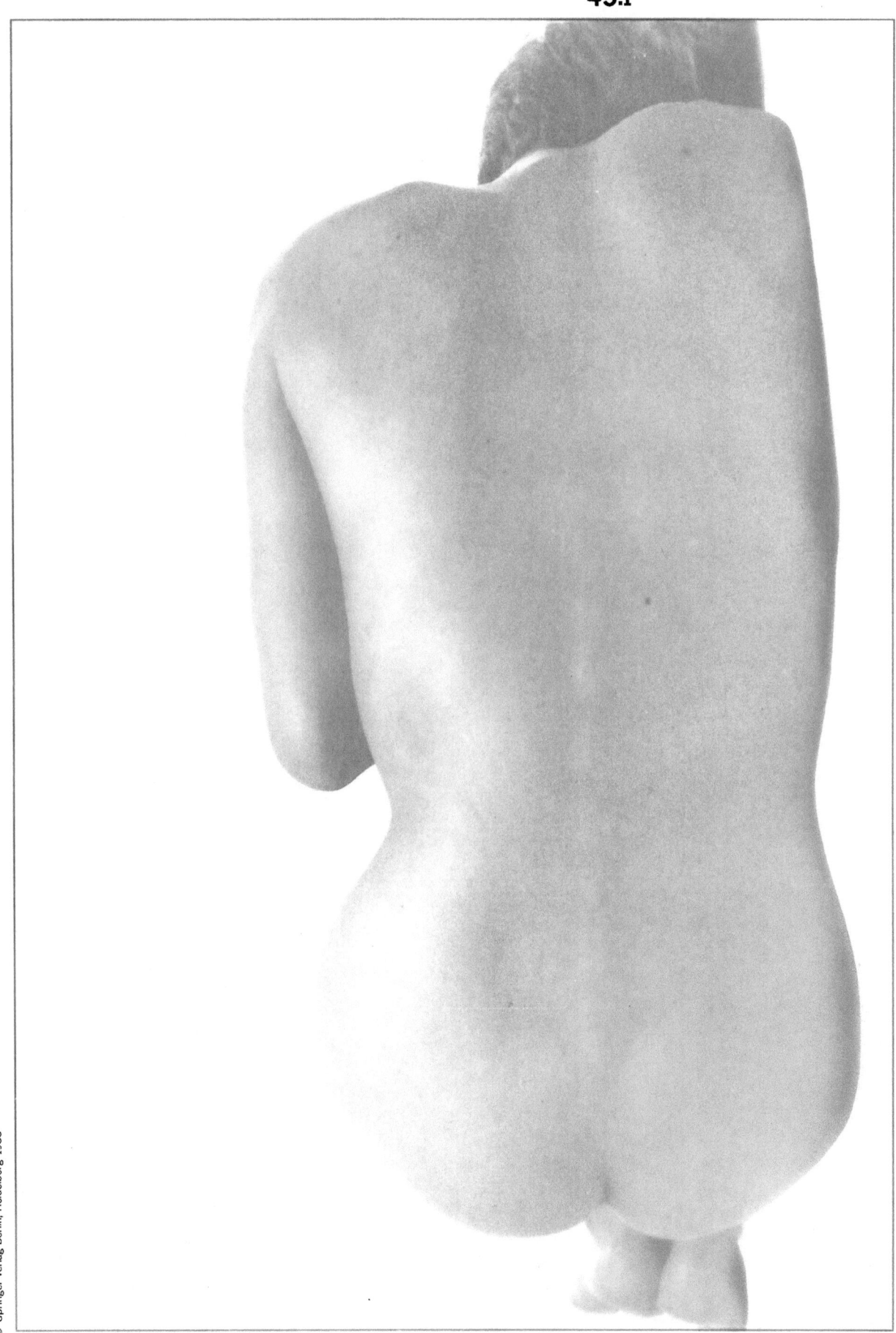

Thoracic Paravertebral Nerve Block

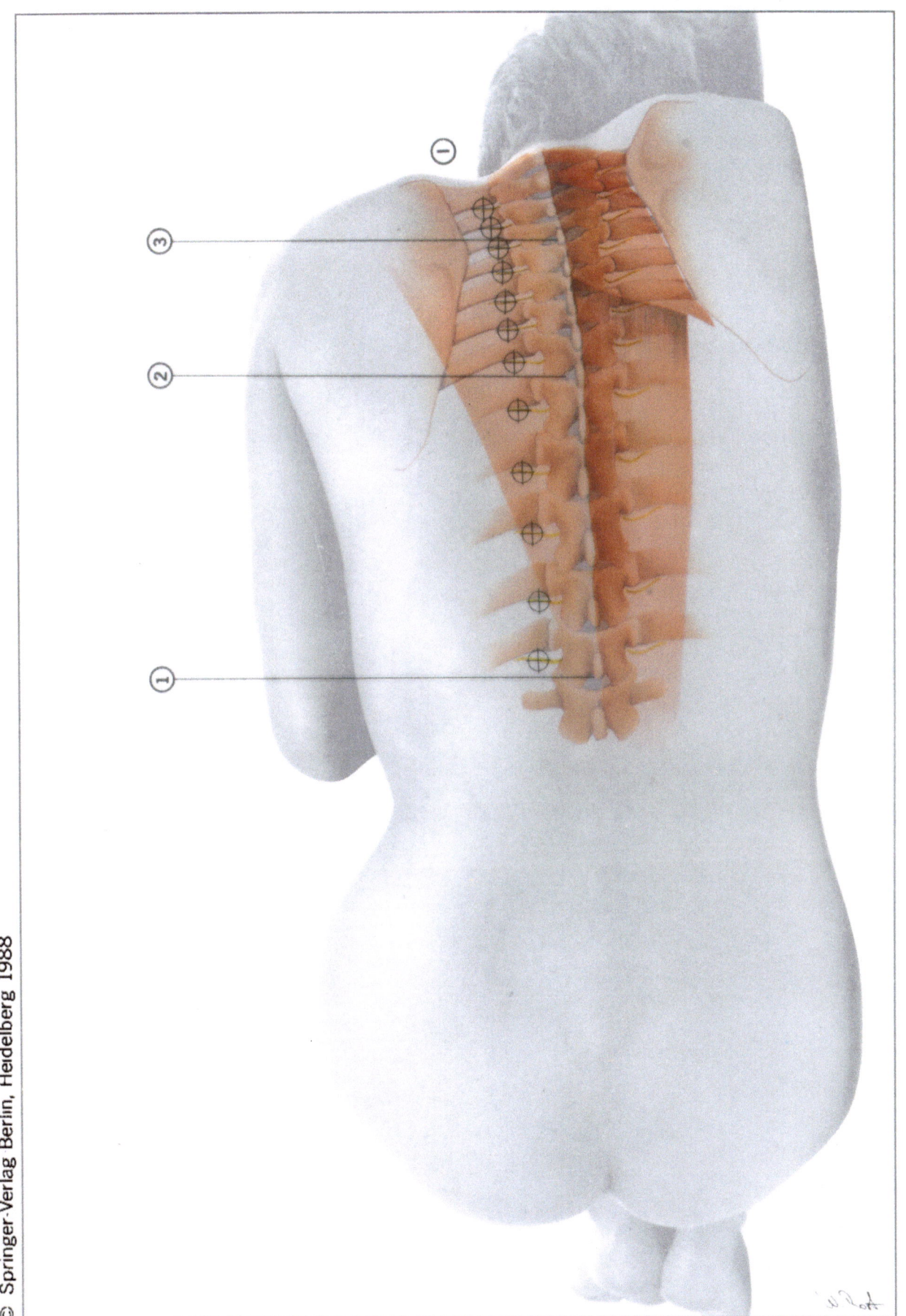

① Injection sites for thoracic paravertebral nerve block (with patient in lateral decubitus position). ① Spinous process of T12. ② T7–8 interspace. ③ Spinous process of T3

①   ①

⊗   ⊗

⊗   ⊗

⊗   ⊗ ————————————————①

⊗   ⊗ ————————————————②

⊗   ⊗ ————————————————③

© Springer-Verlag Berlin, Heidelberg 1988

① Injection sites for lumbar paravertebral nerve block. ① Spinous process of L3. ② Spinous process of L4. ③ Spinous process of L5

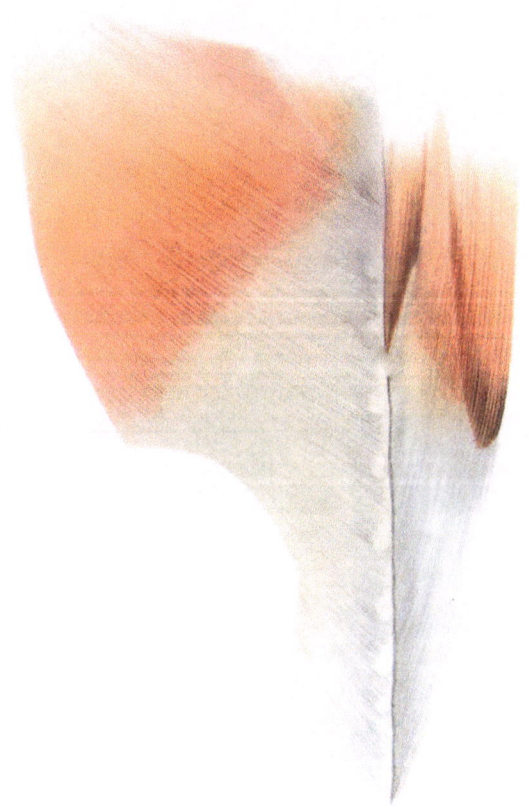

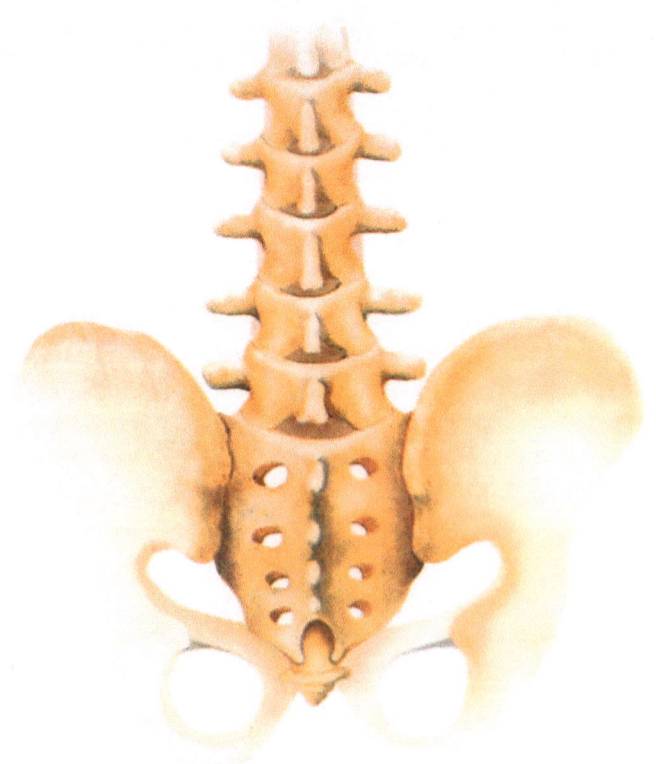

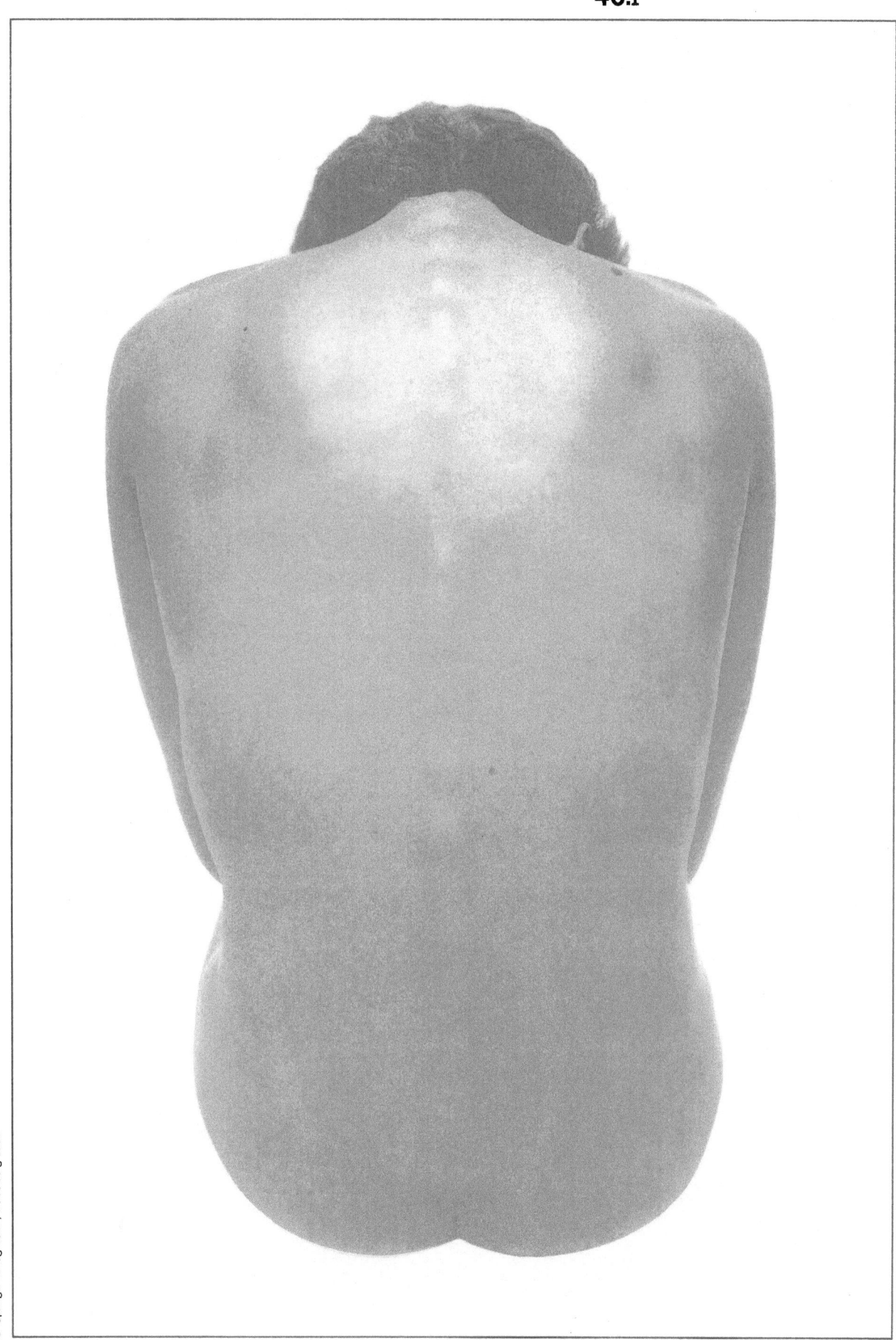

Lumbar Paravertebral Nerve Block

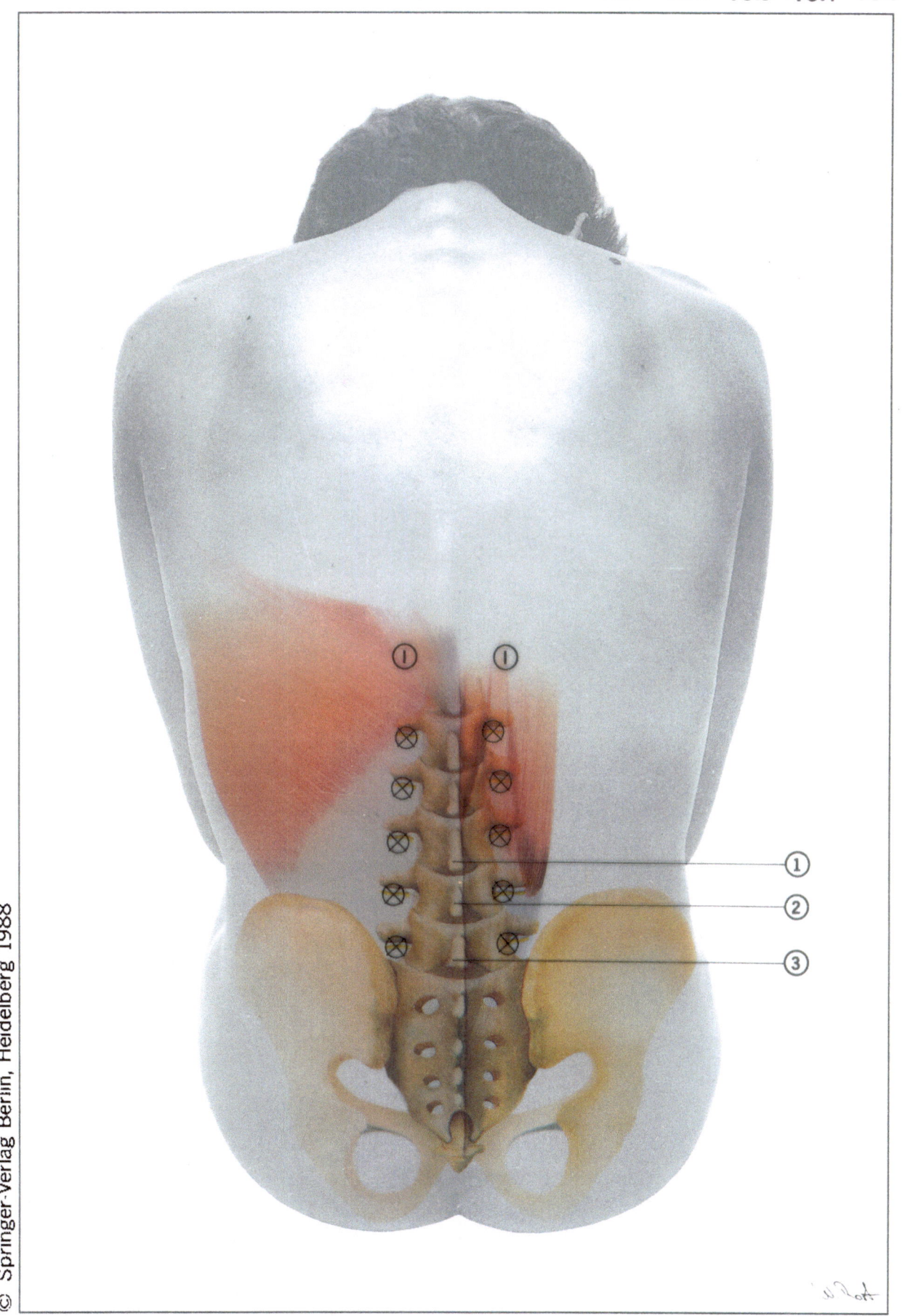

① Injection sites for lumbar paravertebral nerve block. ① Spinous process of L3. ② Spinous process of L4. ③ Spinous process of L5

①—————————— Ⓘ ⊕   ⑤

②—————————— Ⓘ⊕   ————————

③—————————— Ⓘ⊕

④—————————— ⒾⓋ⊕

                                    ——————————————————⑥

                                    ——————————————————⑦

Ⓘ Injection site for S1. Ⓘ Injection site for S2. Ⓘ Injection site for S3. Ⓘ Injection site for S4. ① First sacral foramen. ② Second sacral foramen. ③ Third sacral foramen. ④ Fourth sacral foramen. ⑤ Posterior superior iliac spine. ⑥ Sacral hiatus. ⑦ Sacral cornu

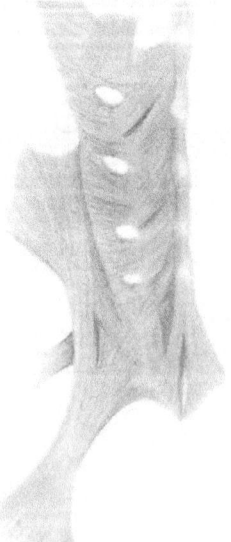

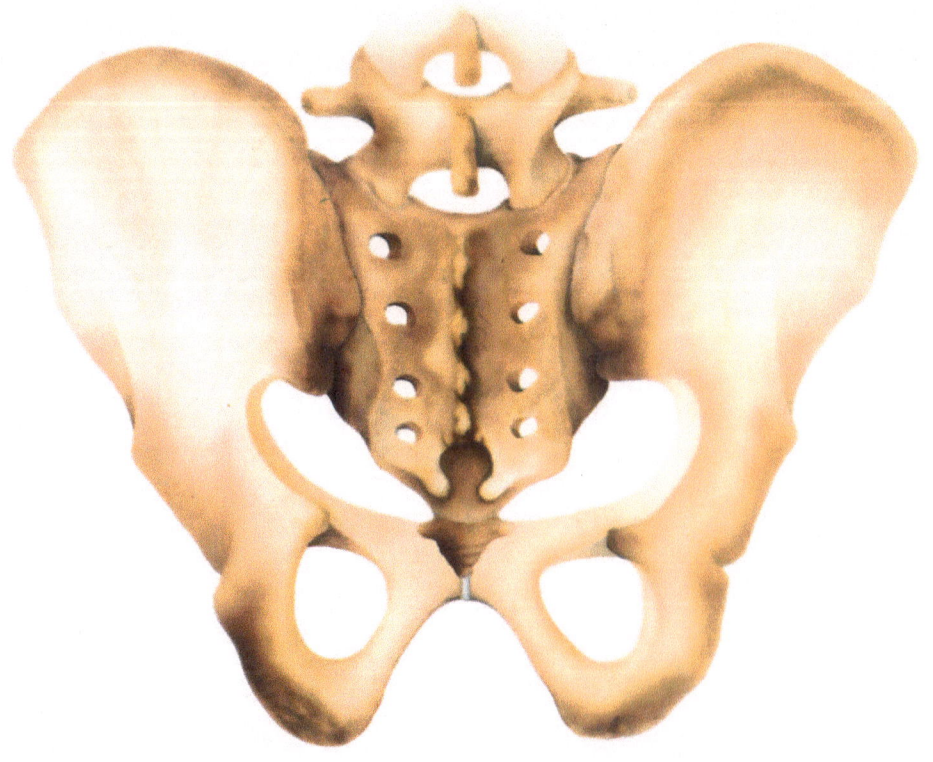

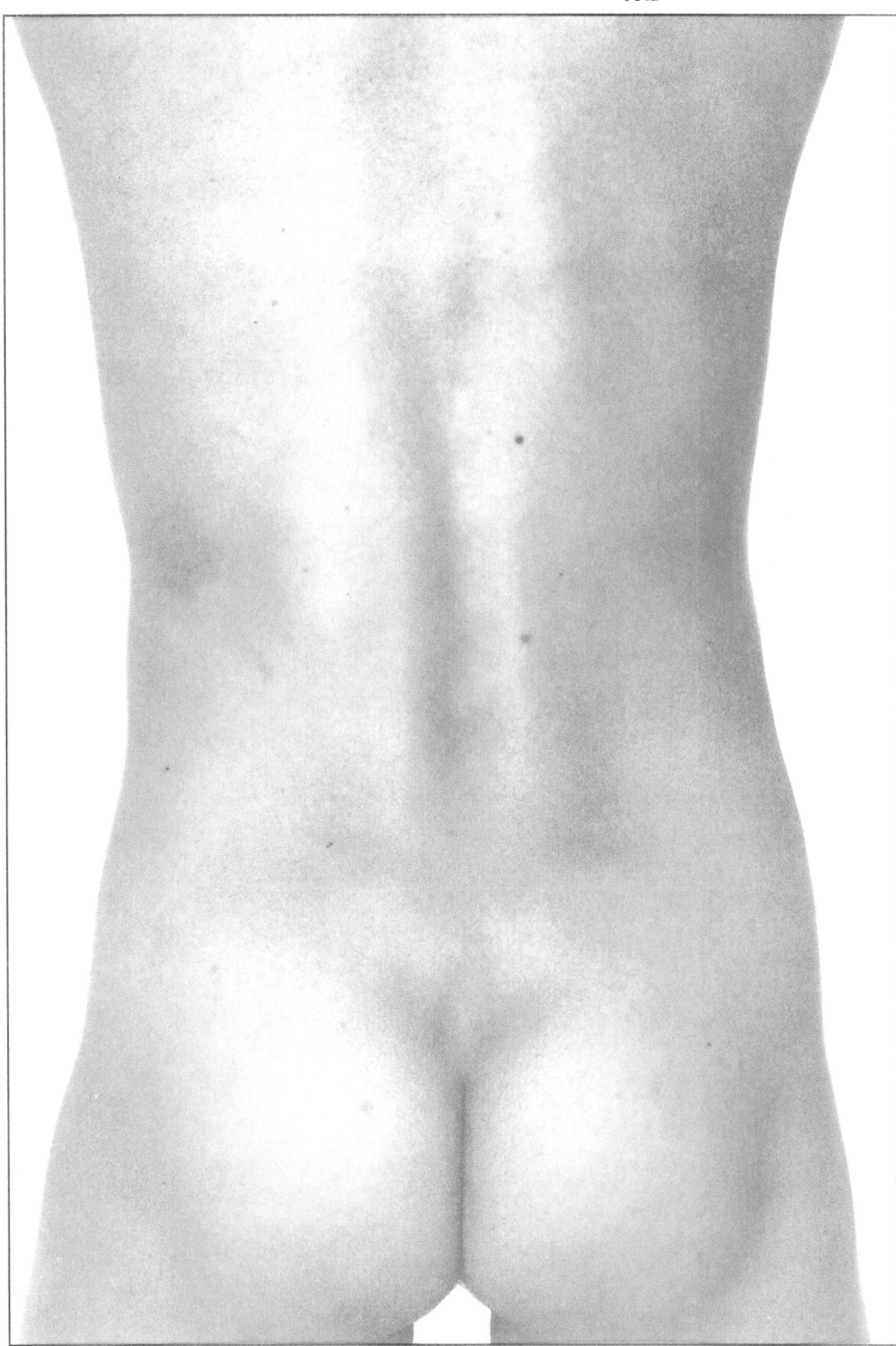

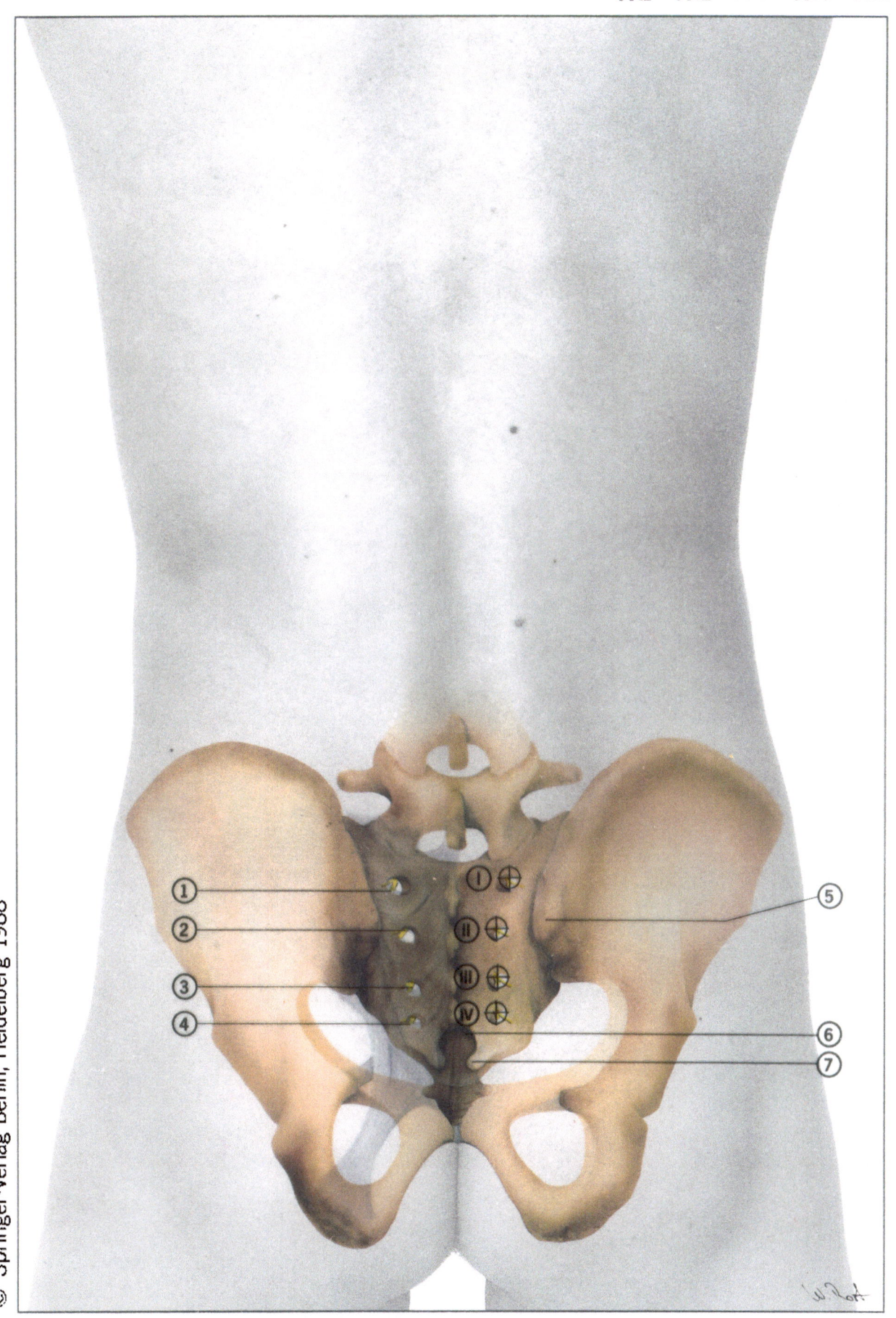

① Injection site for S1. ② Injection site for S2. ③ Injection site for S3. ④ Injection site for S4. ① First sacral foramen. ② Second sacral foramen.
③ Third sacral foramen. ④ Fourth sacral foramen. ⑤ Posterior superior iliac spine. ⑥ Sacral hiatus. ⑦ Sacral cornu

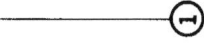

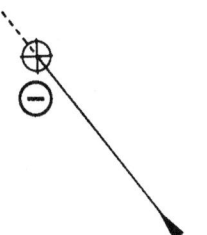

© Springer-Verlag Berlin, Heidelberg 1988

① Injection site and angulation of needle in the transperineal approach for pudendal nerve block. ① Ischial tuberosity

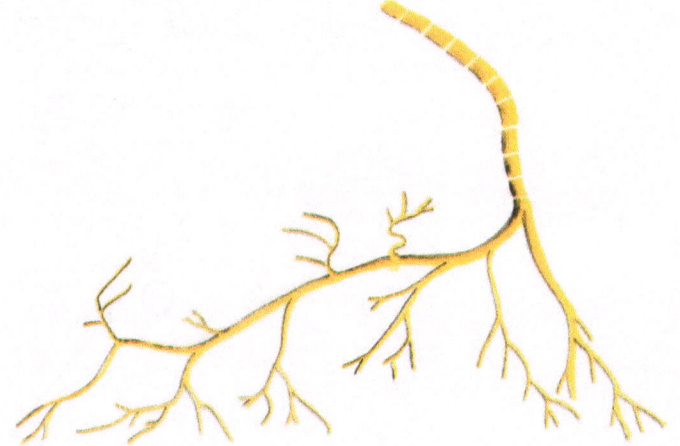

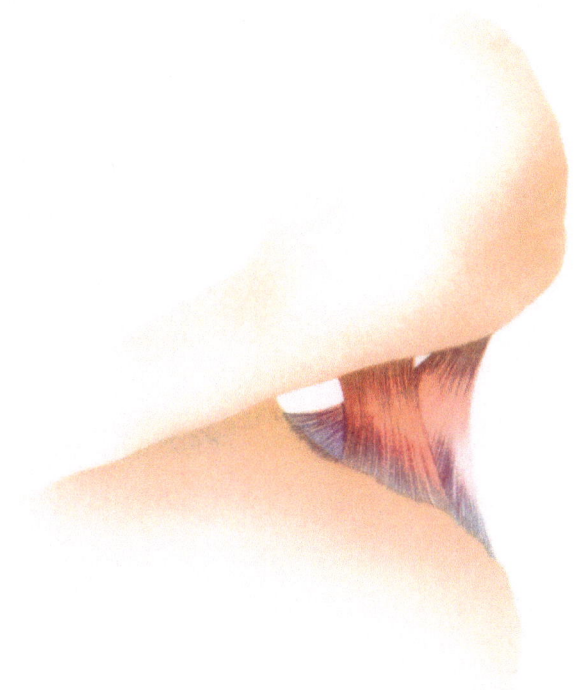

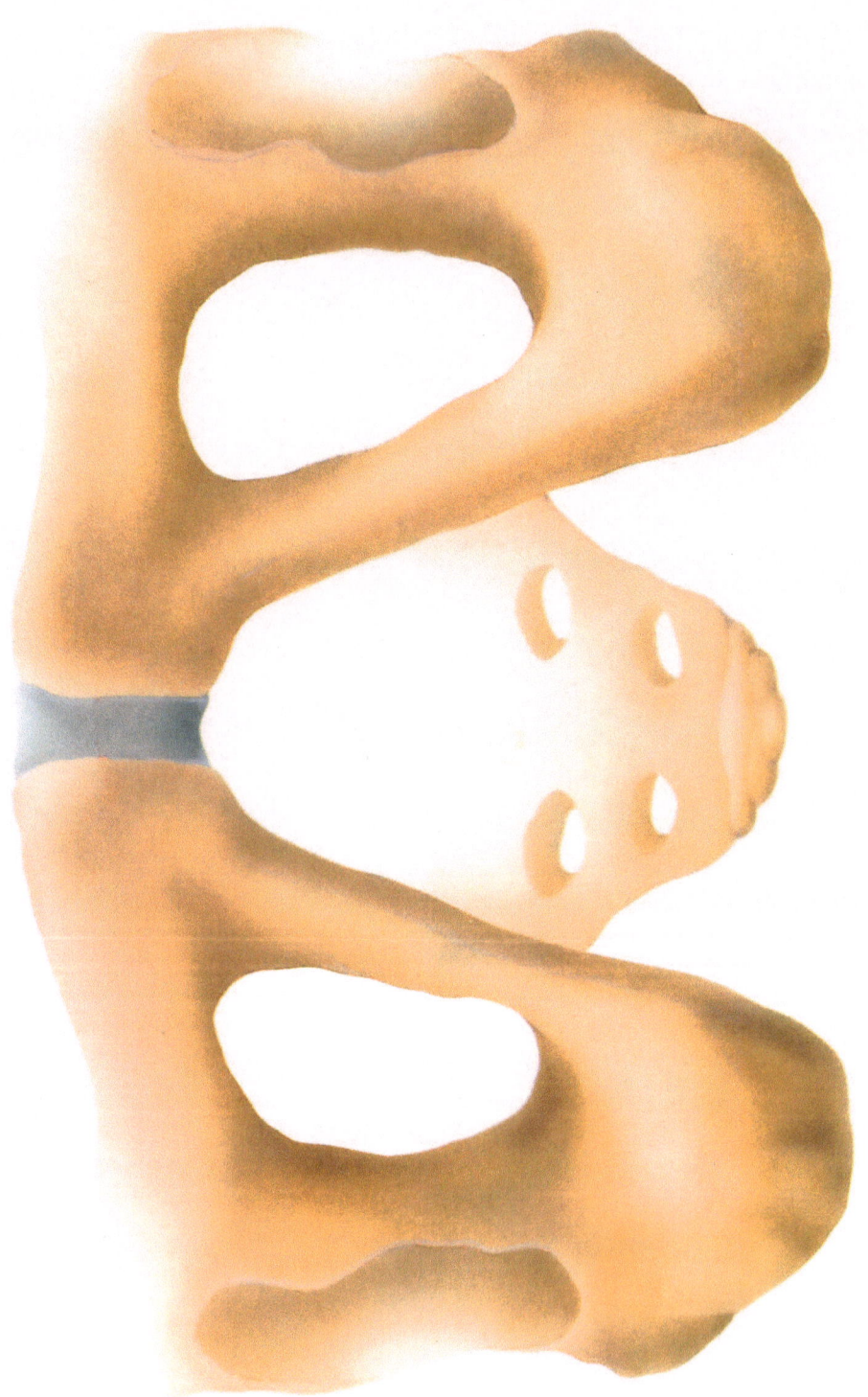

48.1

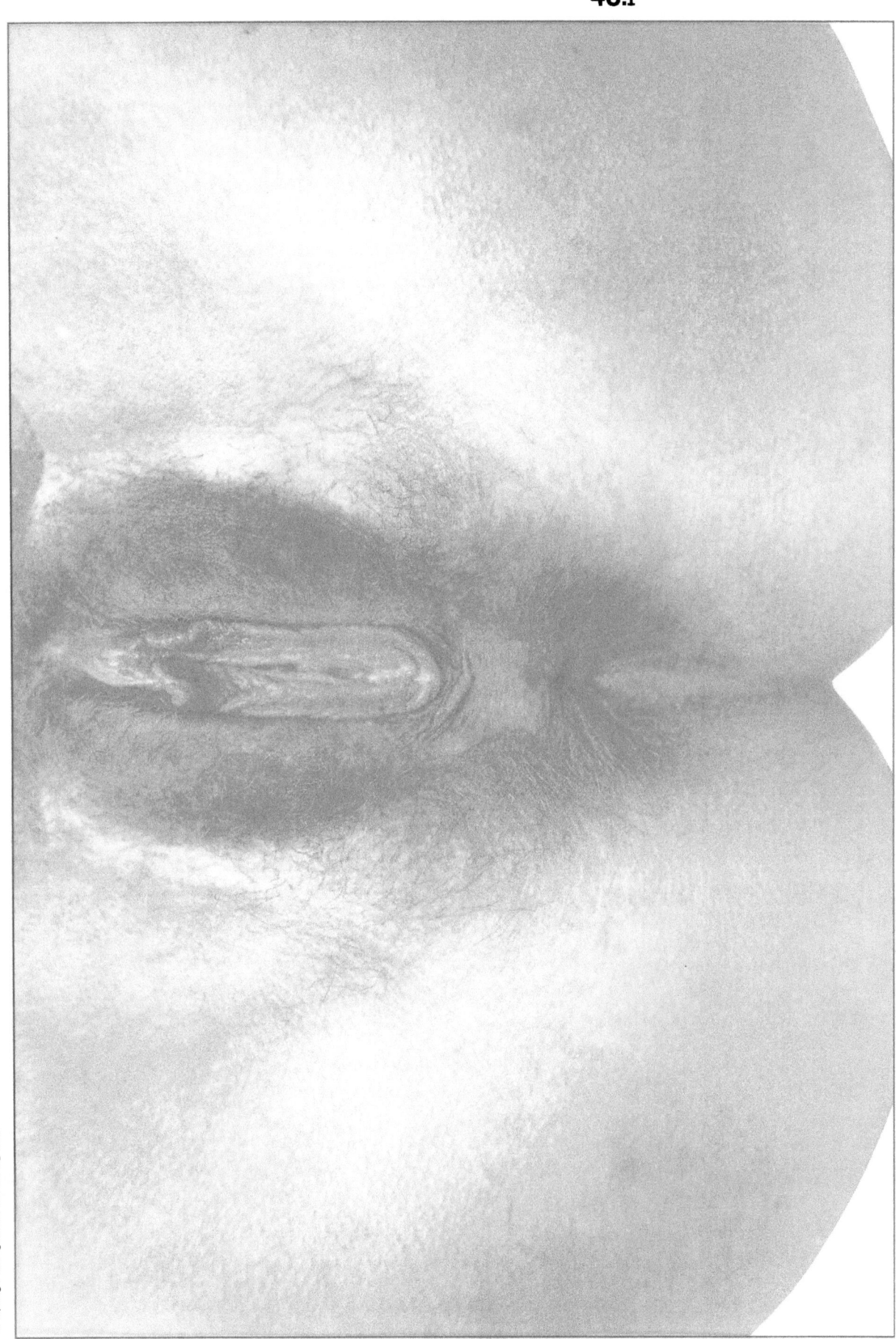

Pudendal Nerve Block: Transperineal Approach

Pudendal Nerve Block: Transperineal Approach

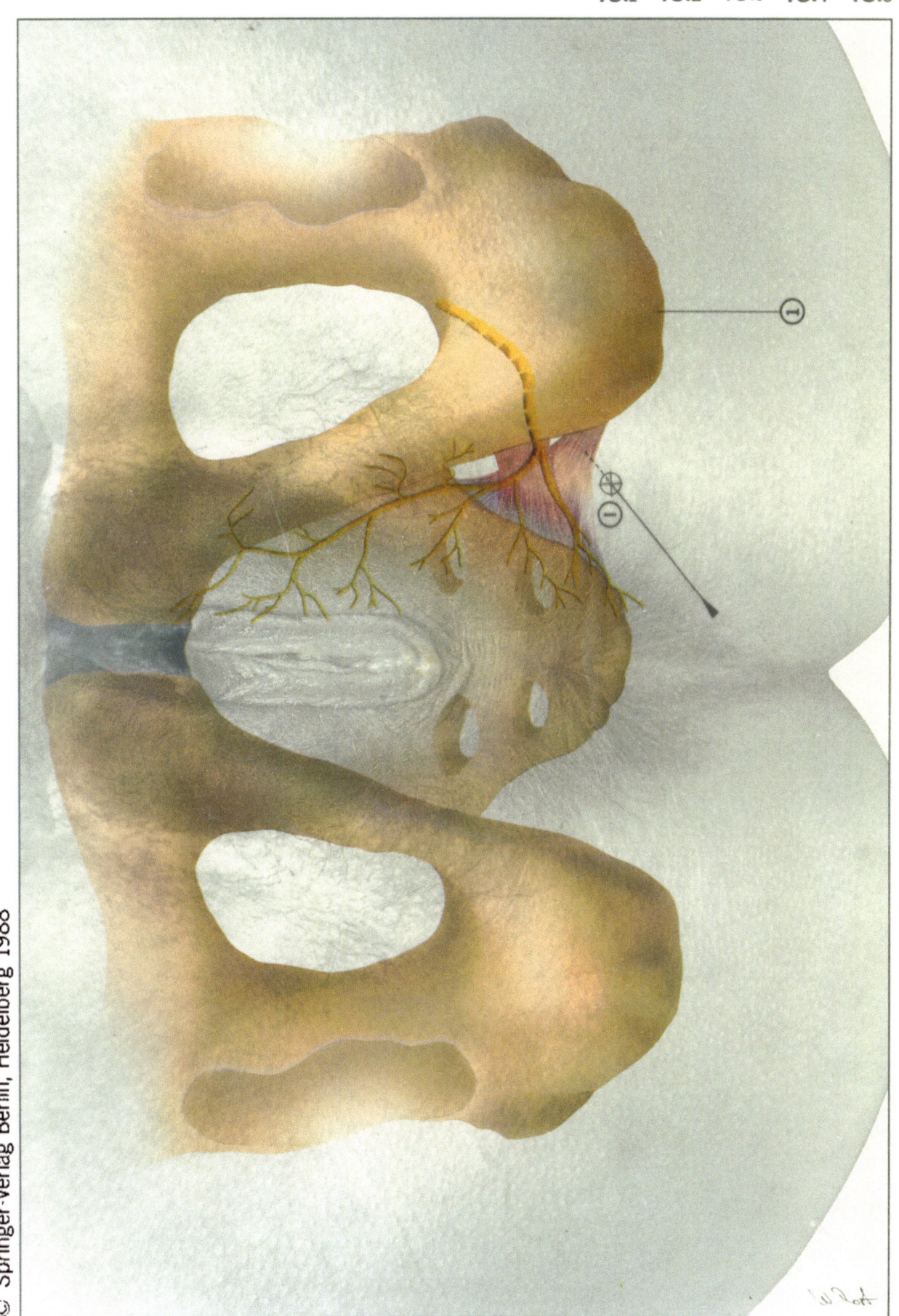

① Injection site and angulation of needle in the transperineal approach for pudendal nerve block. ① Ischial tuberosity

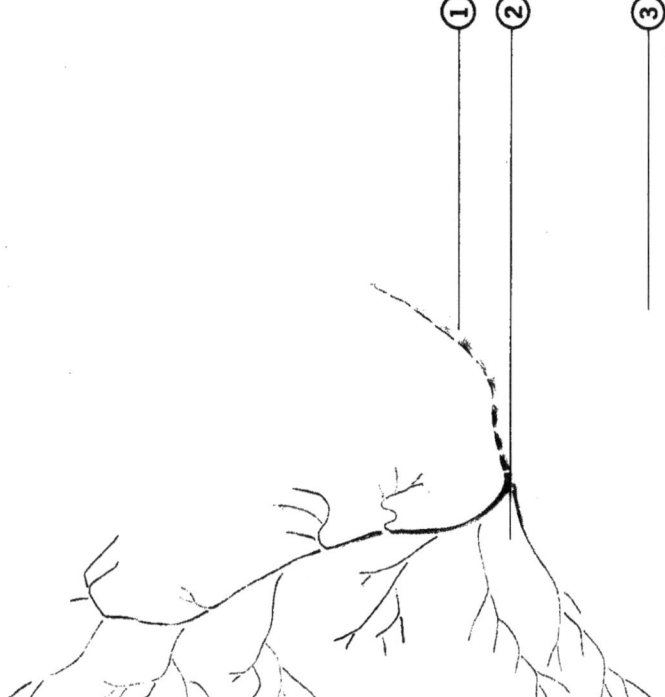

① Position of the pudendal nerve behind the ischial ramus in Alcock's canal. ② Sacrospinous ligament. ③ Ischial tuberosity

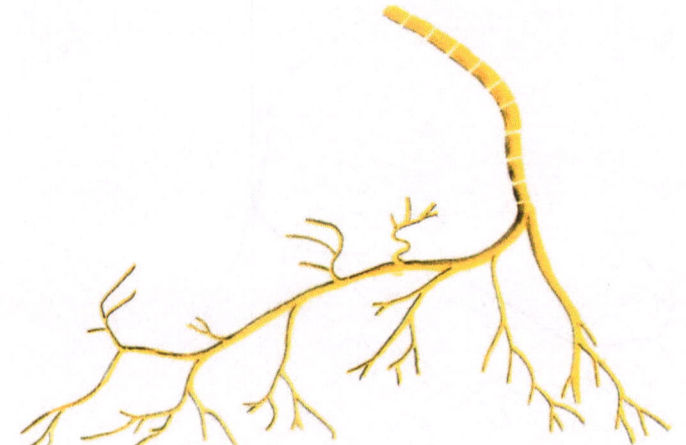

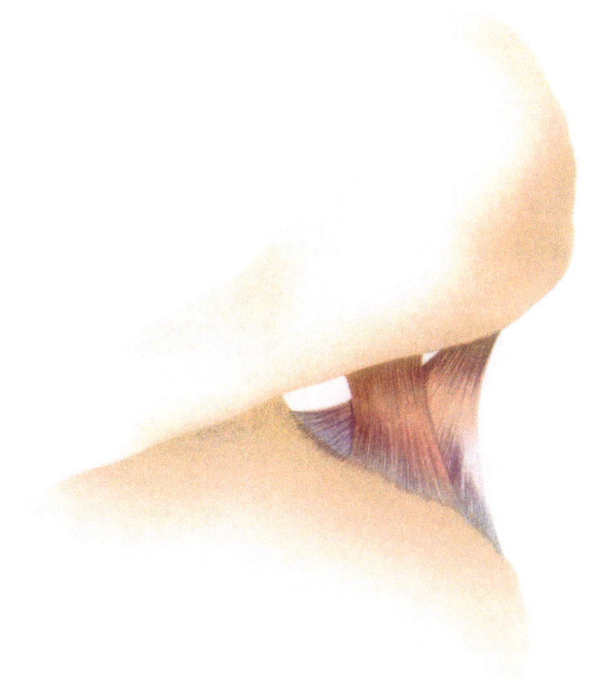

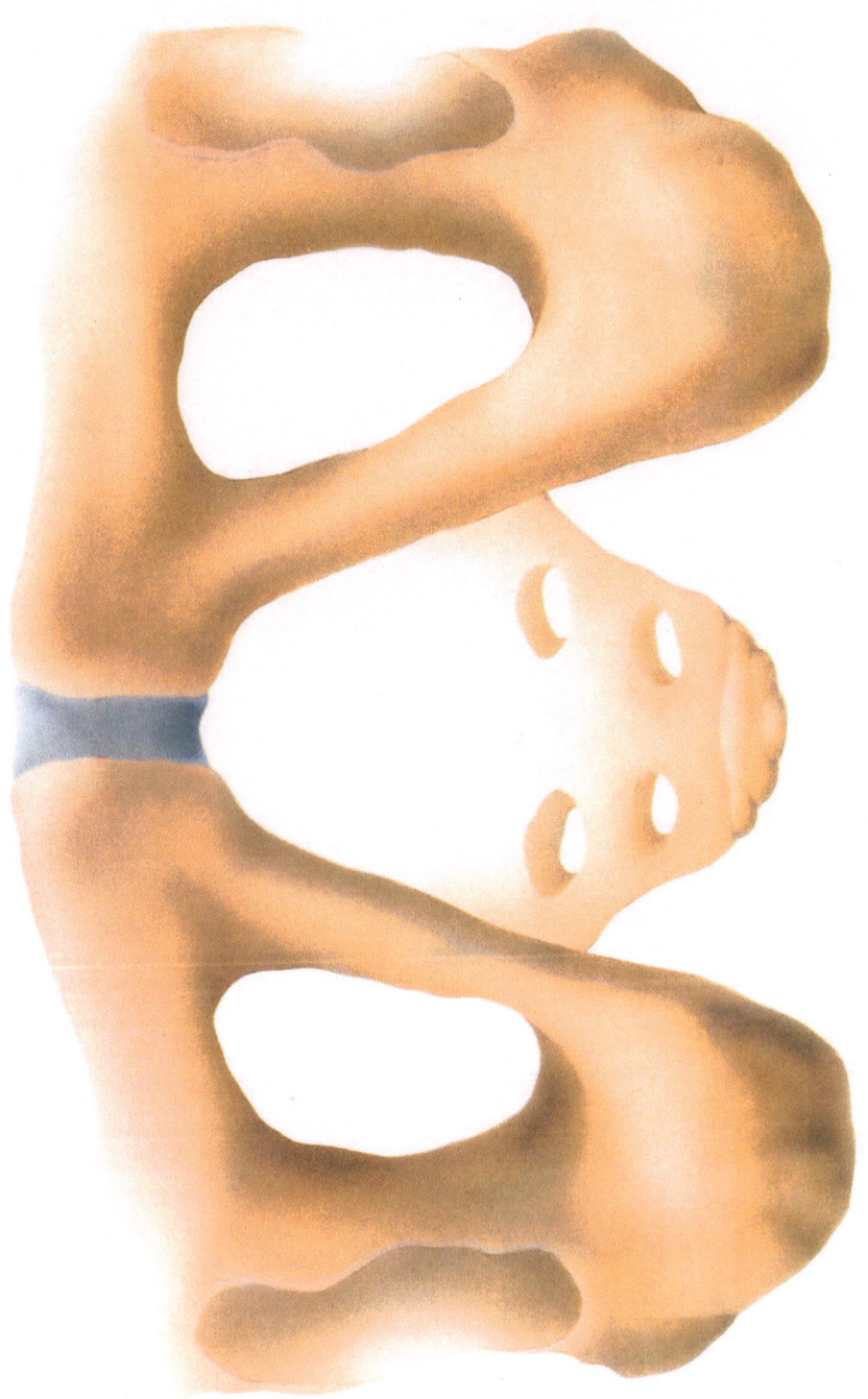

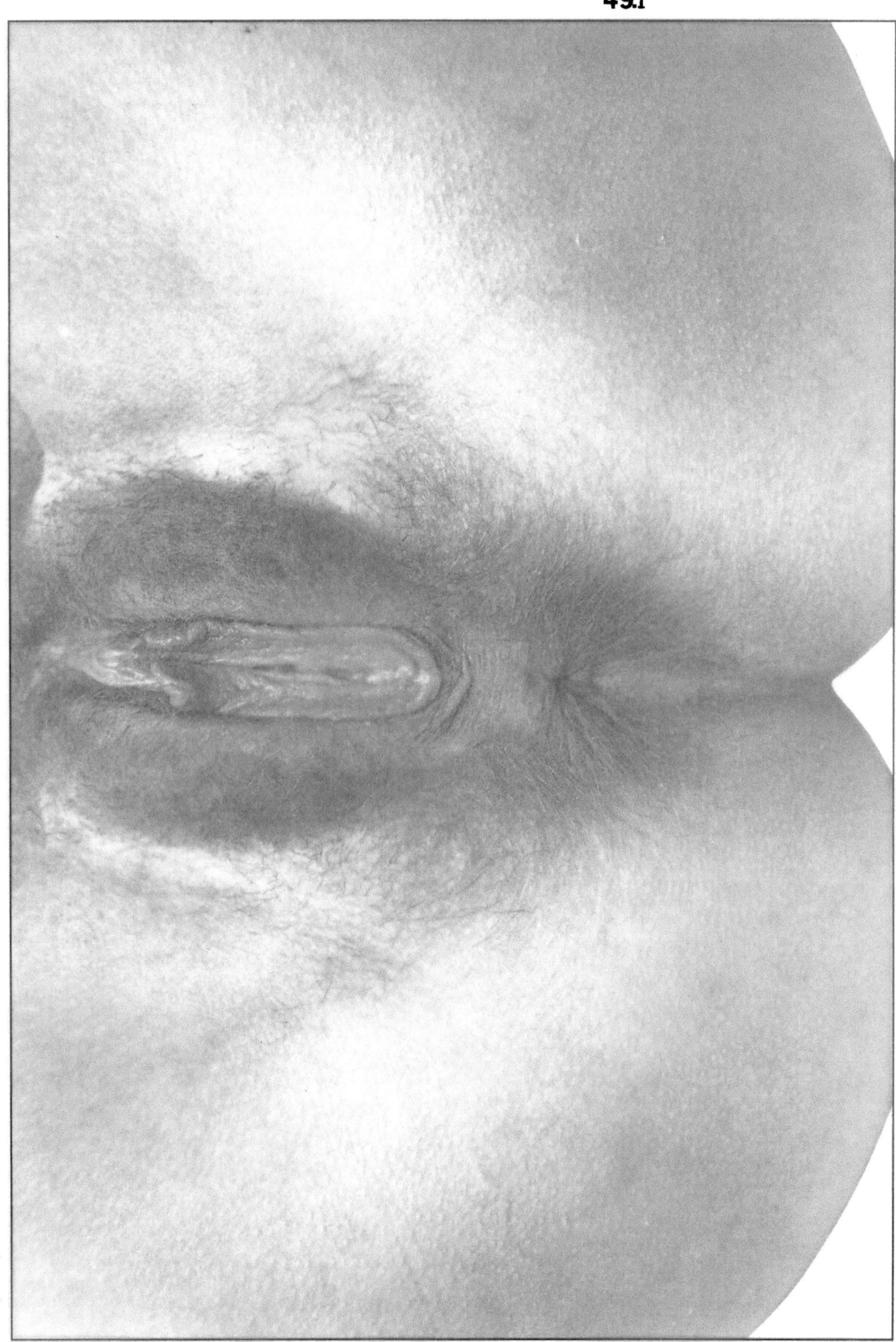

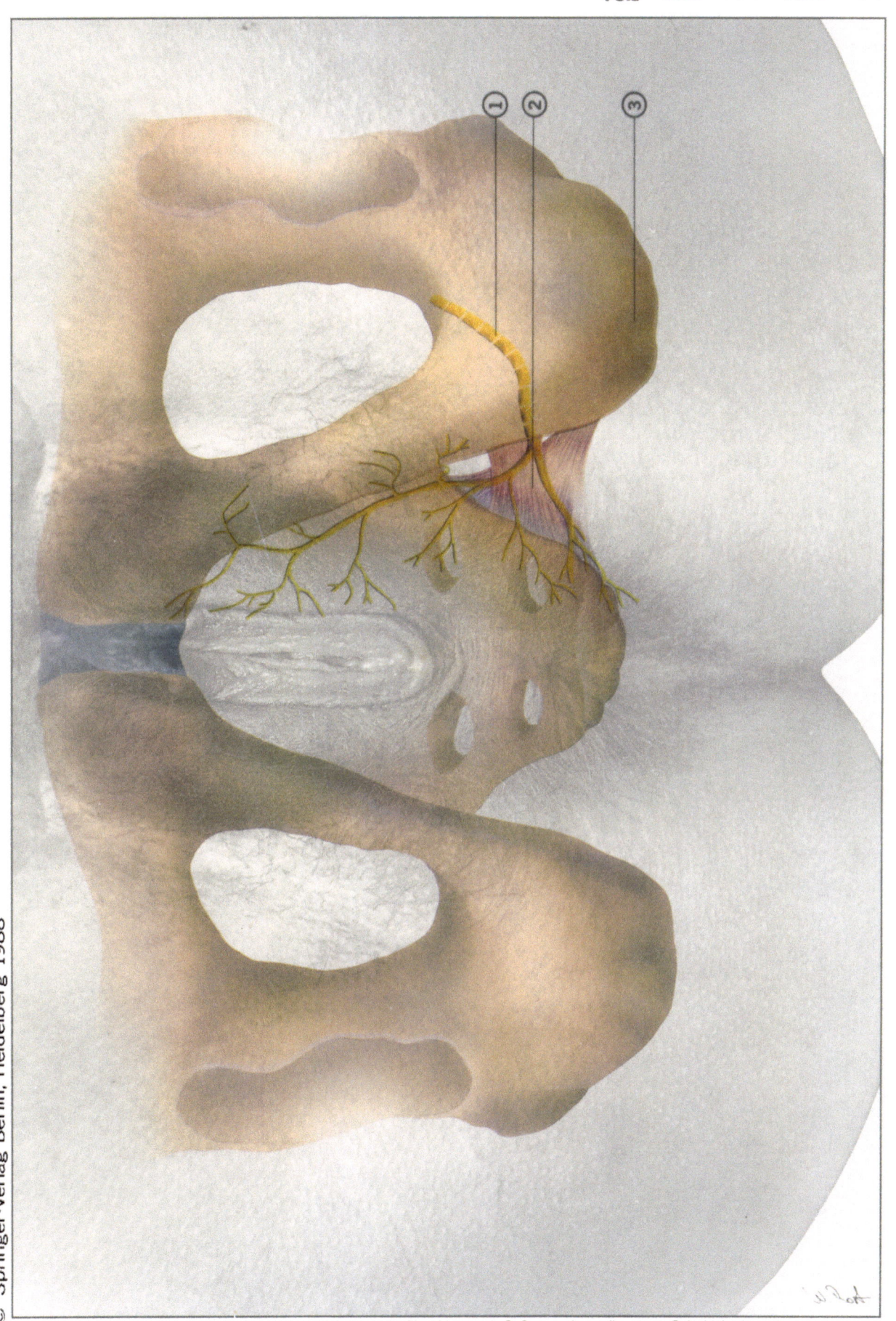

① Position of the pudendal nerve behind the ischial ramus in Alcock's canal. ② Sacrospinous ligament. ③ Ischial tuberosity

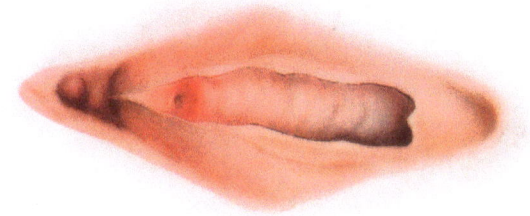

Perineum

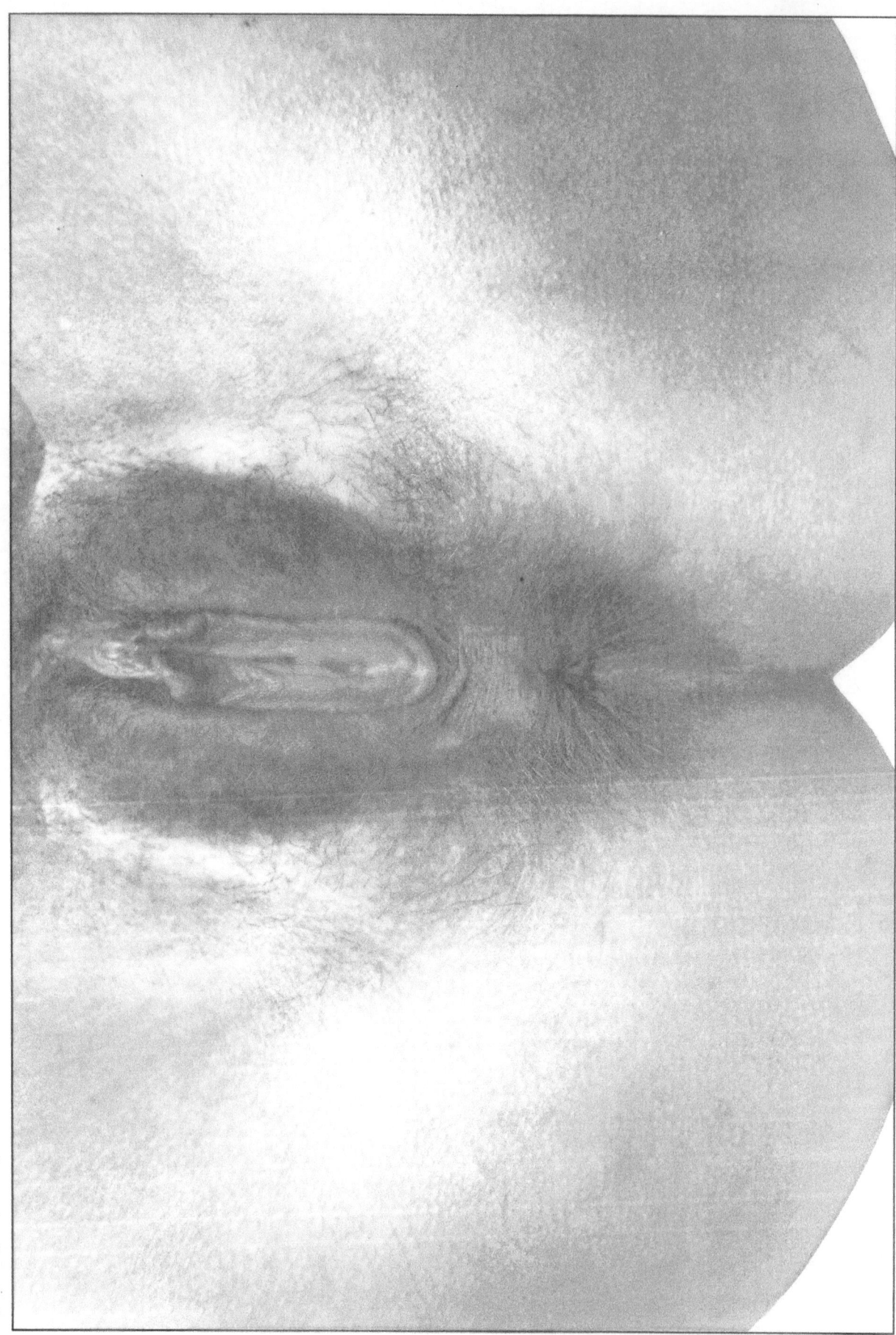

50

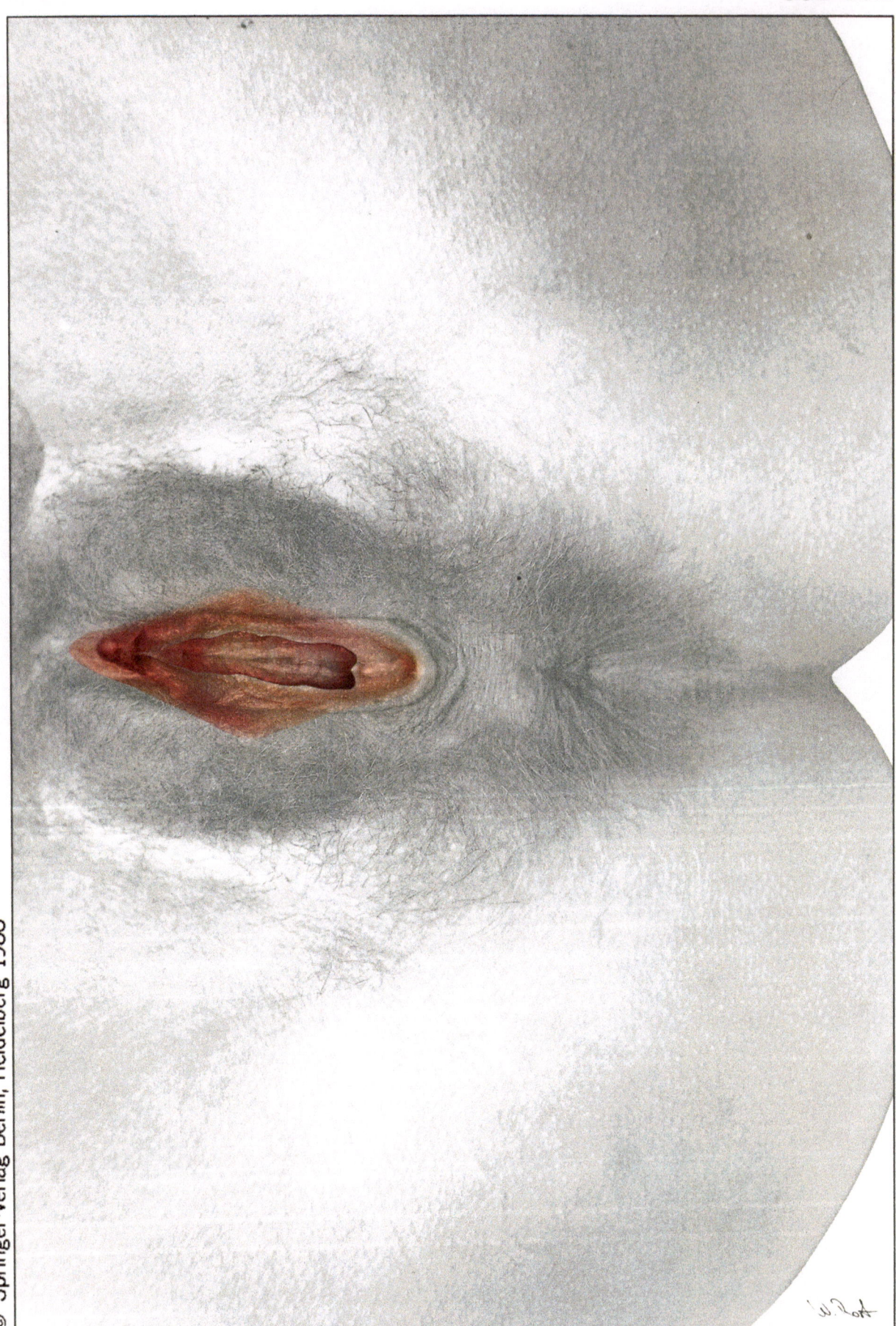

Perineum

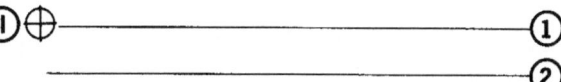

① Injection site for sacrococcygeal nerve block. ① Sacral hiatus. ② Sacrococcygeal nerve

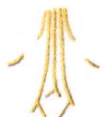

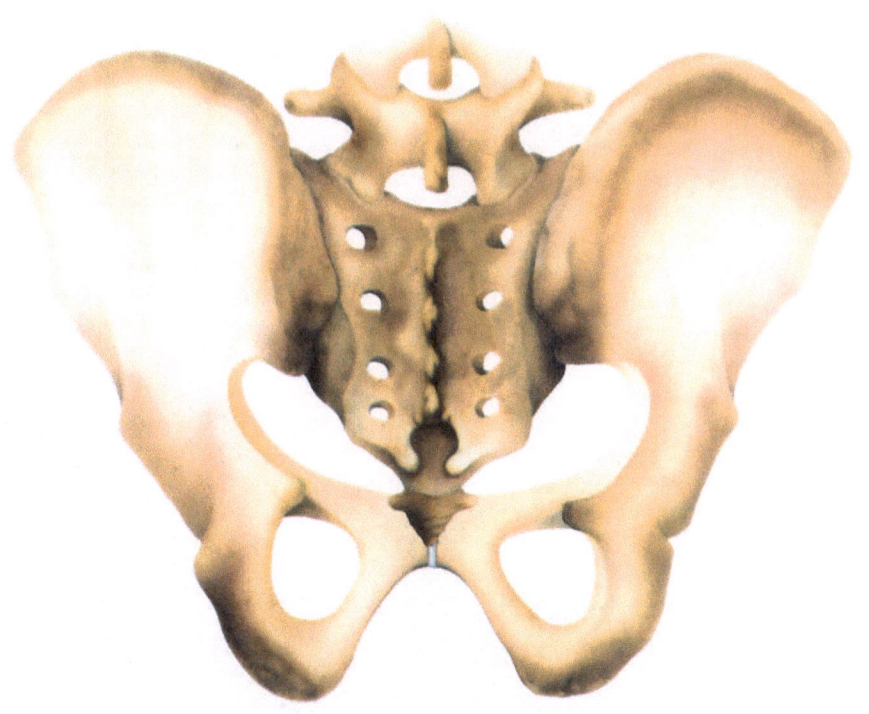

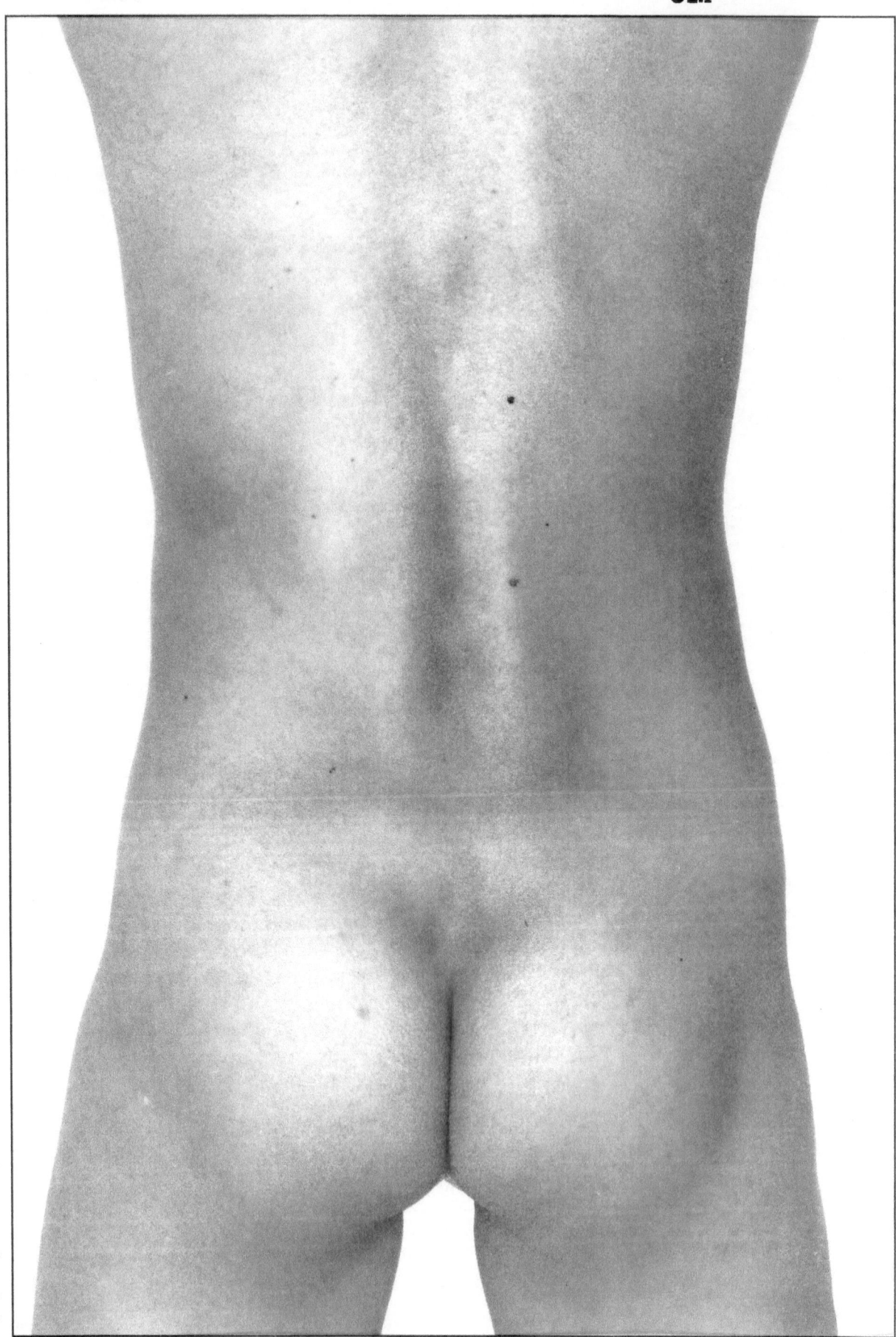

Sacrococcygeal Plexus Block

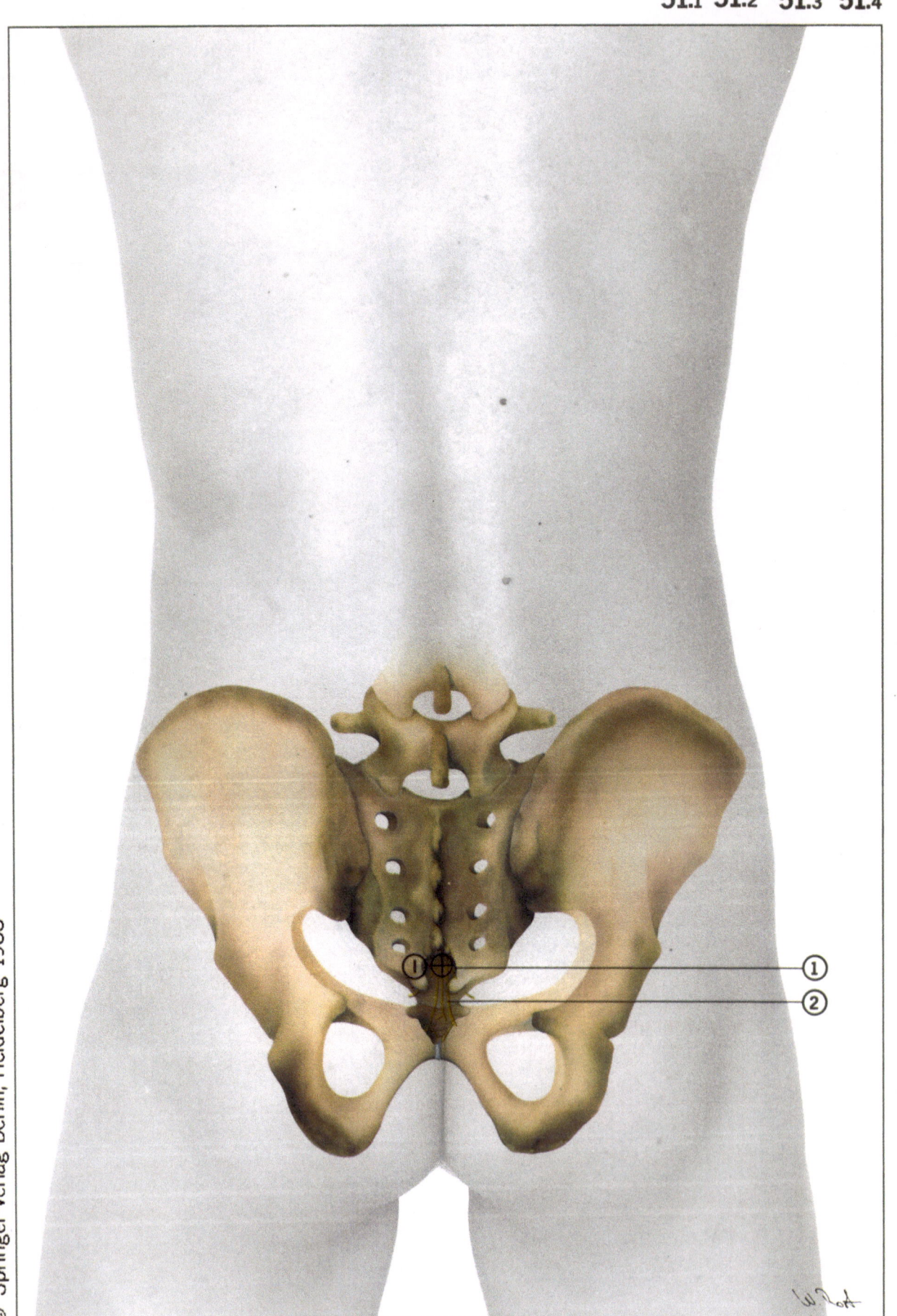

① Injection site for sacrococcygeal nerve block. ① Sacral hiatus. ② Sacrococcygeal nerve

① Injection sites for stellate ganglion block (anterior approach). ① Common carotid artery. ② Internal jugular vein. ③ Stellate ganglion (at level of C7 – T1). ④ Sternocleidomastoid muscle. ⑤ Cricoid cartilage

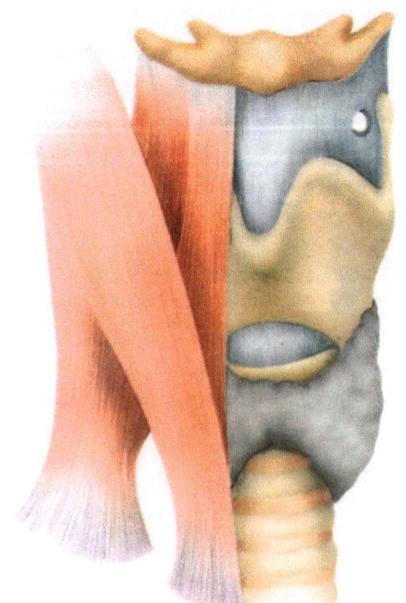

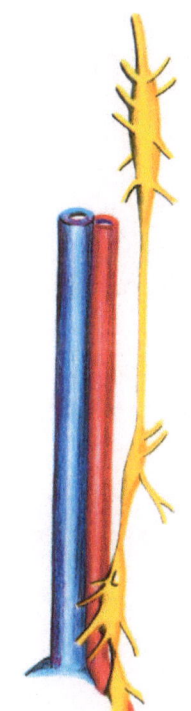

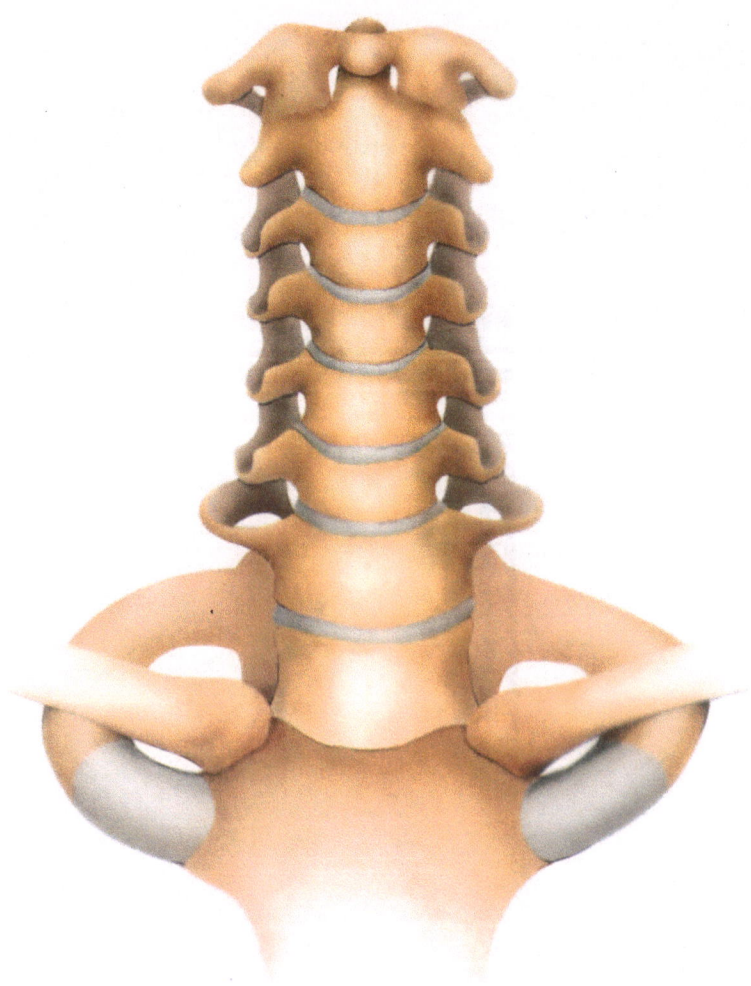

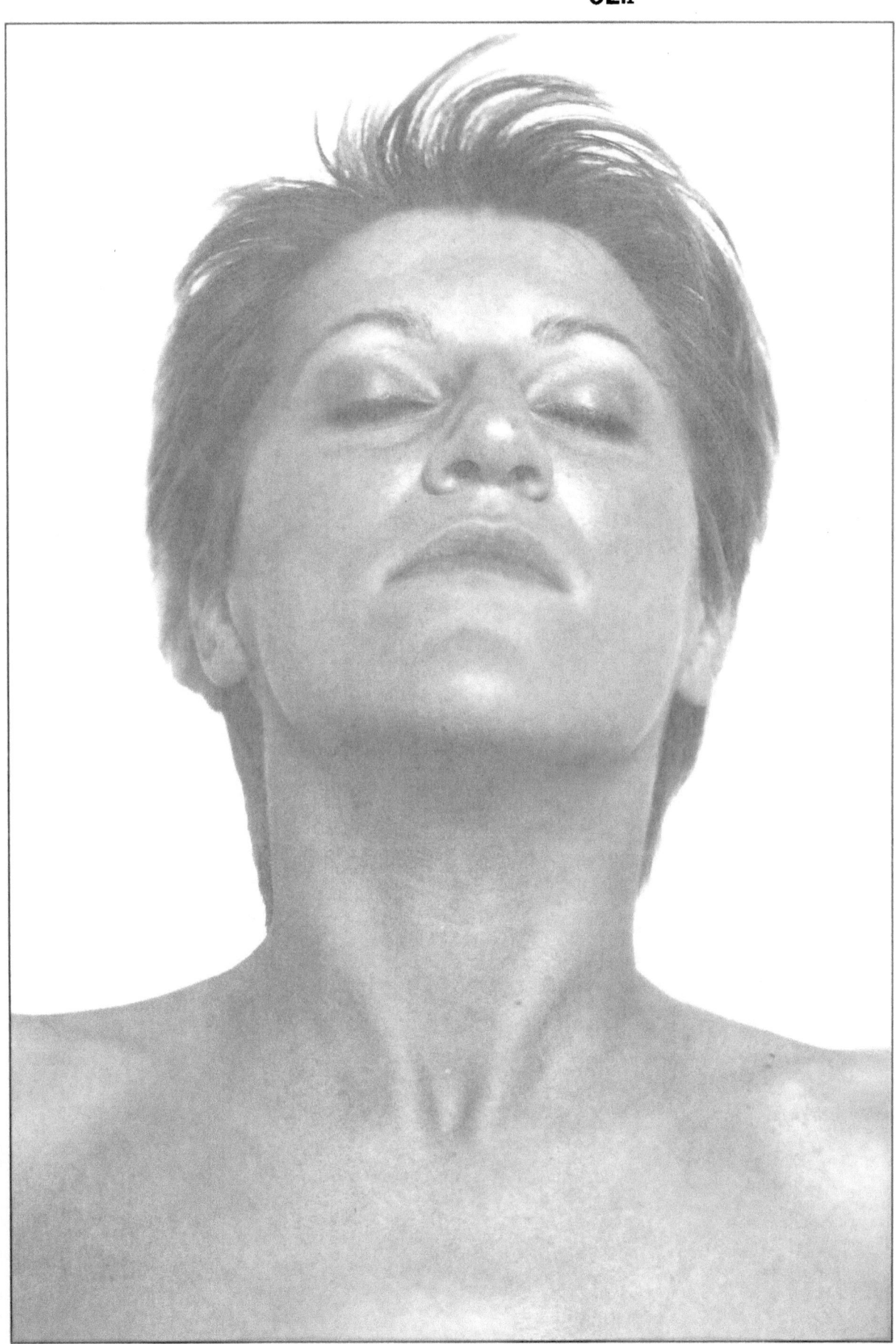

Stellate Ganglion Block: Anterior Approach

52

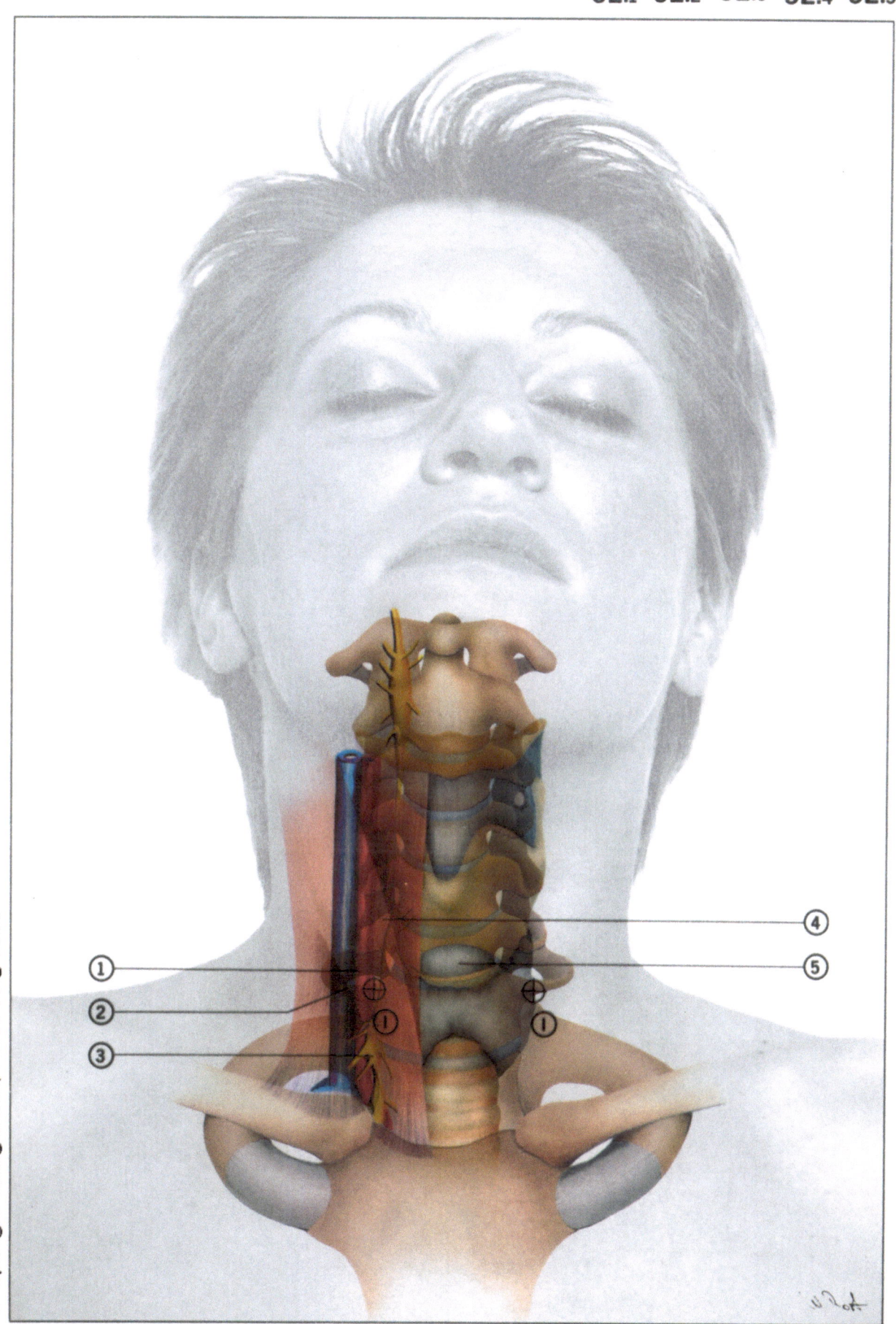

① Injection sites for stellate ganglion block (anterior approach). ① Common carotid artery. ② Internal jugular vein. ③ Stellate ganglion (at level of C7 – T1). ④ Sternocleidomastoid muscle. ⑤ Cricoid cartilage

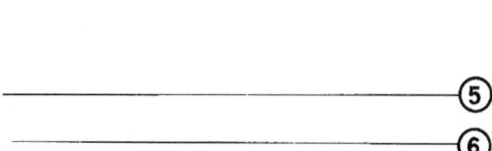

① Point of entry for lateral approach to stellate ganglion block with needle directed toward T1. ⑪ Point of entry for lateral approach with needle directed toward C7. ① Common carotid artery. ② Internal jugular vein. ③ Clavicle. ④ Stellate ganglion. ⑤ Body of C7. ⑥ Body of T1

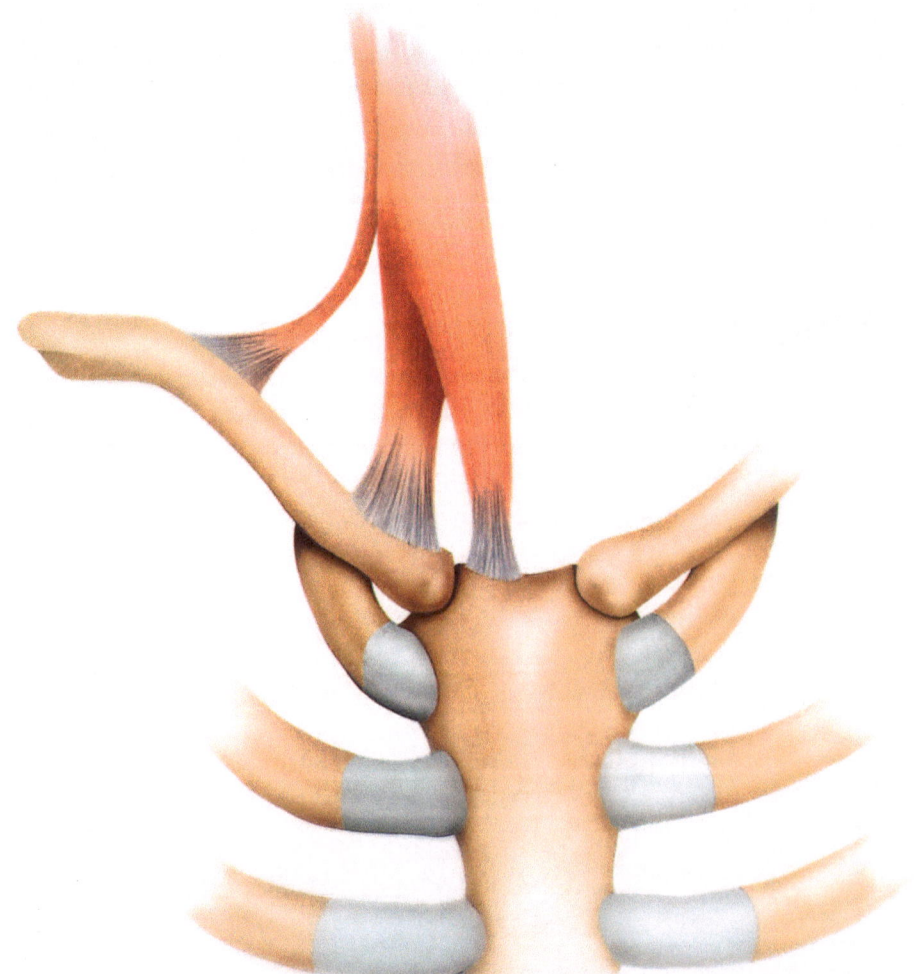

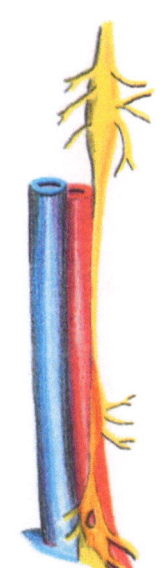

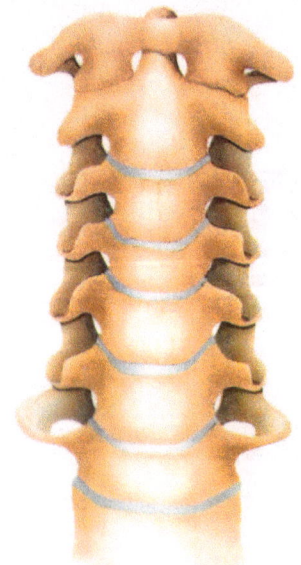

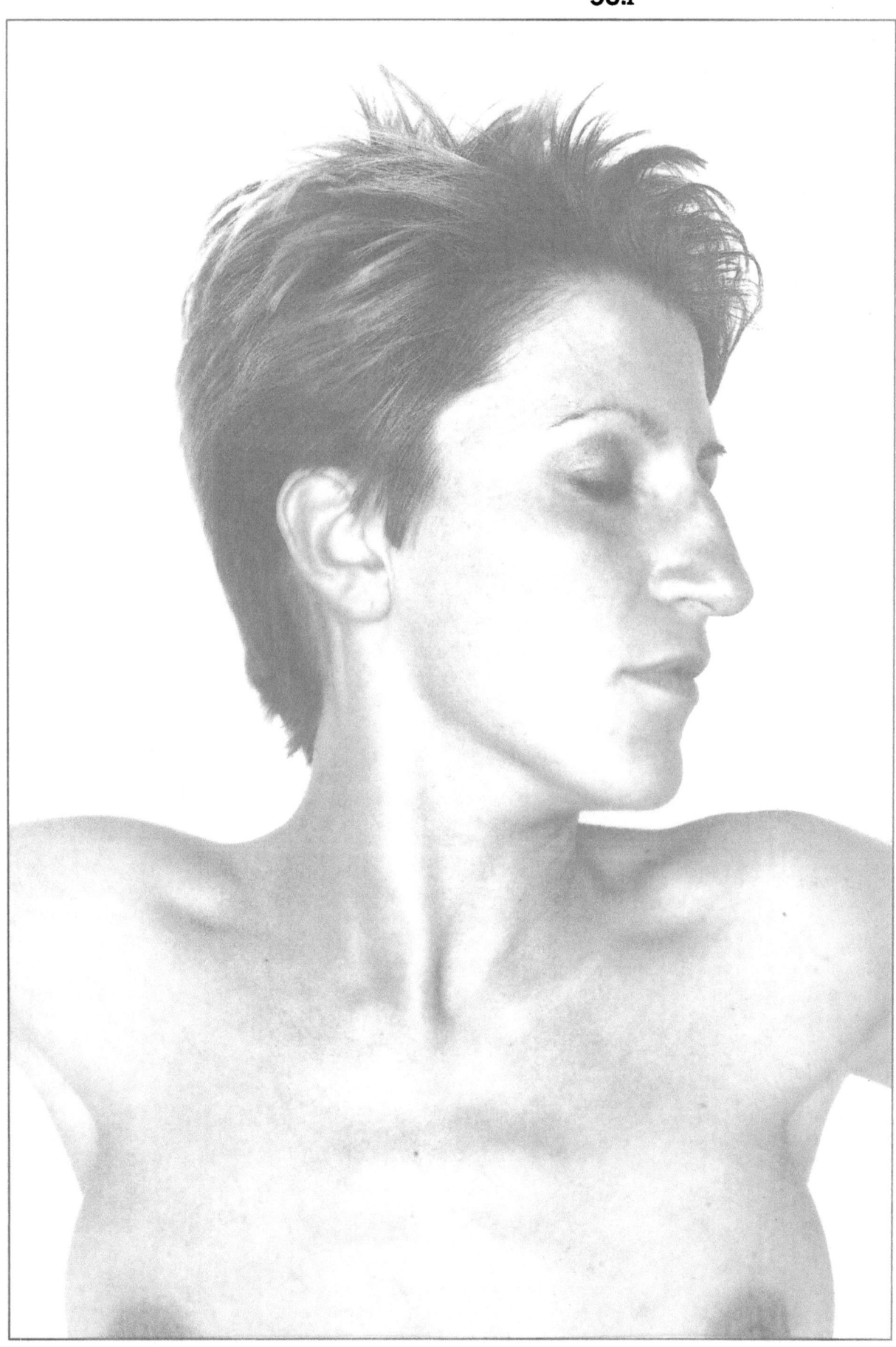

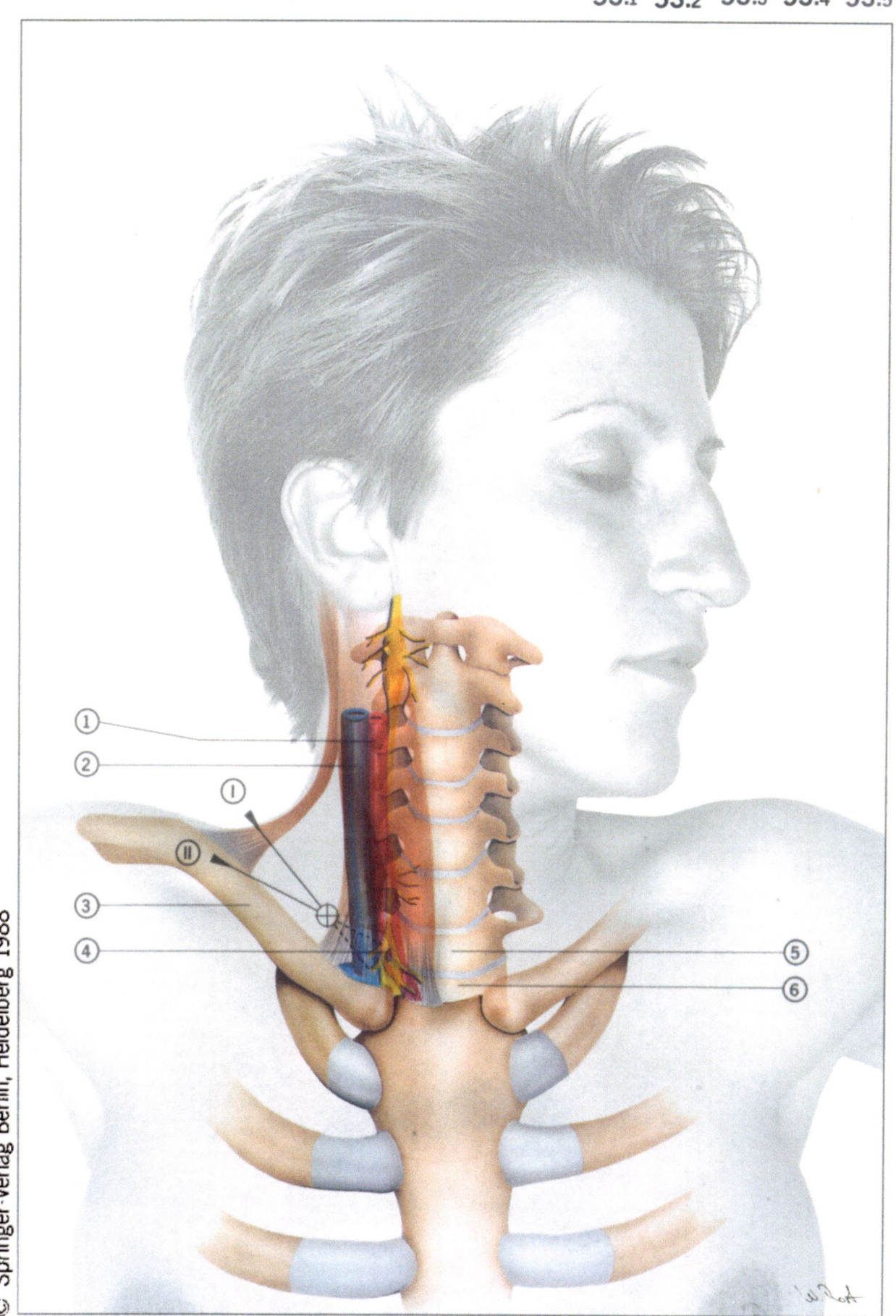

① Point of entry for lateral approach to stellate ganglion block with needle directed toward T1. ⓘ Point of entry for lateral approach with needle directed toward C7. ① Common carotid artery. ② Internal jugular vein. ③ Clavicle. ④ Stellate ganglion. ⑤ Body of C7. ⑥ Body of T1

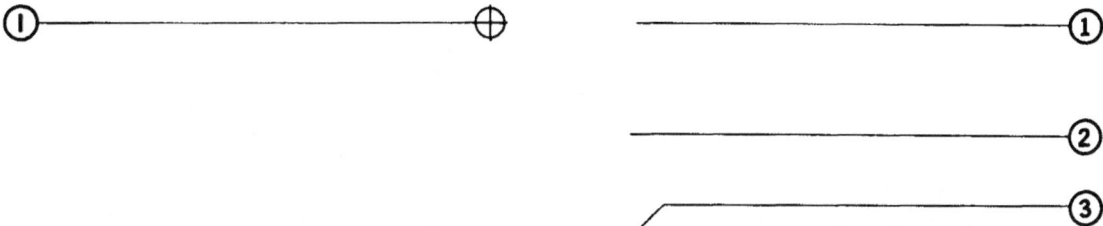

① Injection site for sympathetic block at T6. ① Transverse process of T6. ② Sympathetic trunk. ③ Head of 9th rib

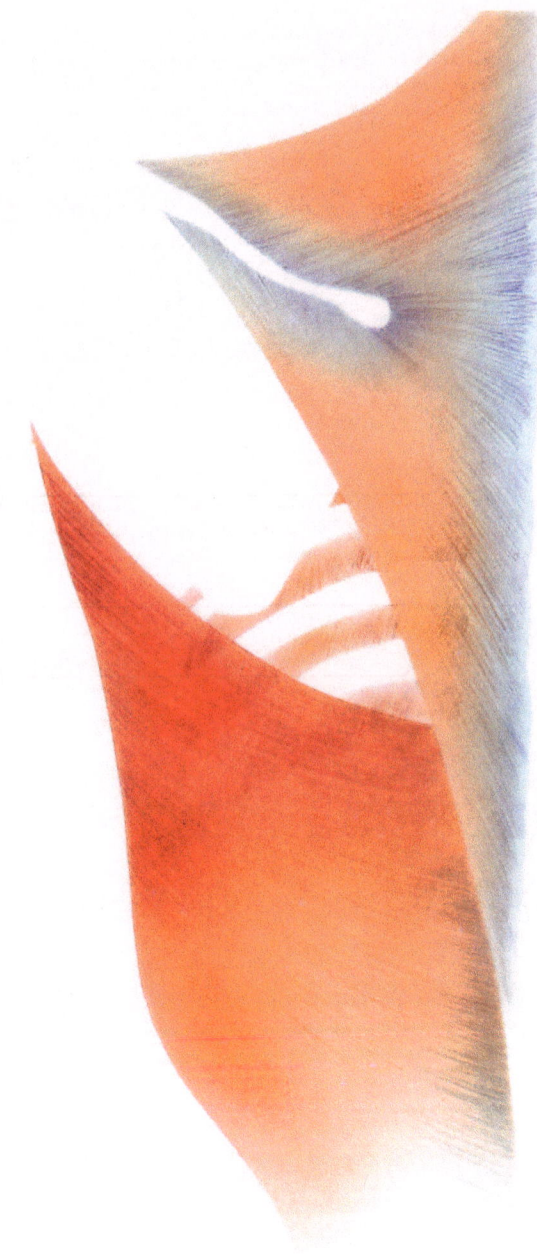

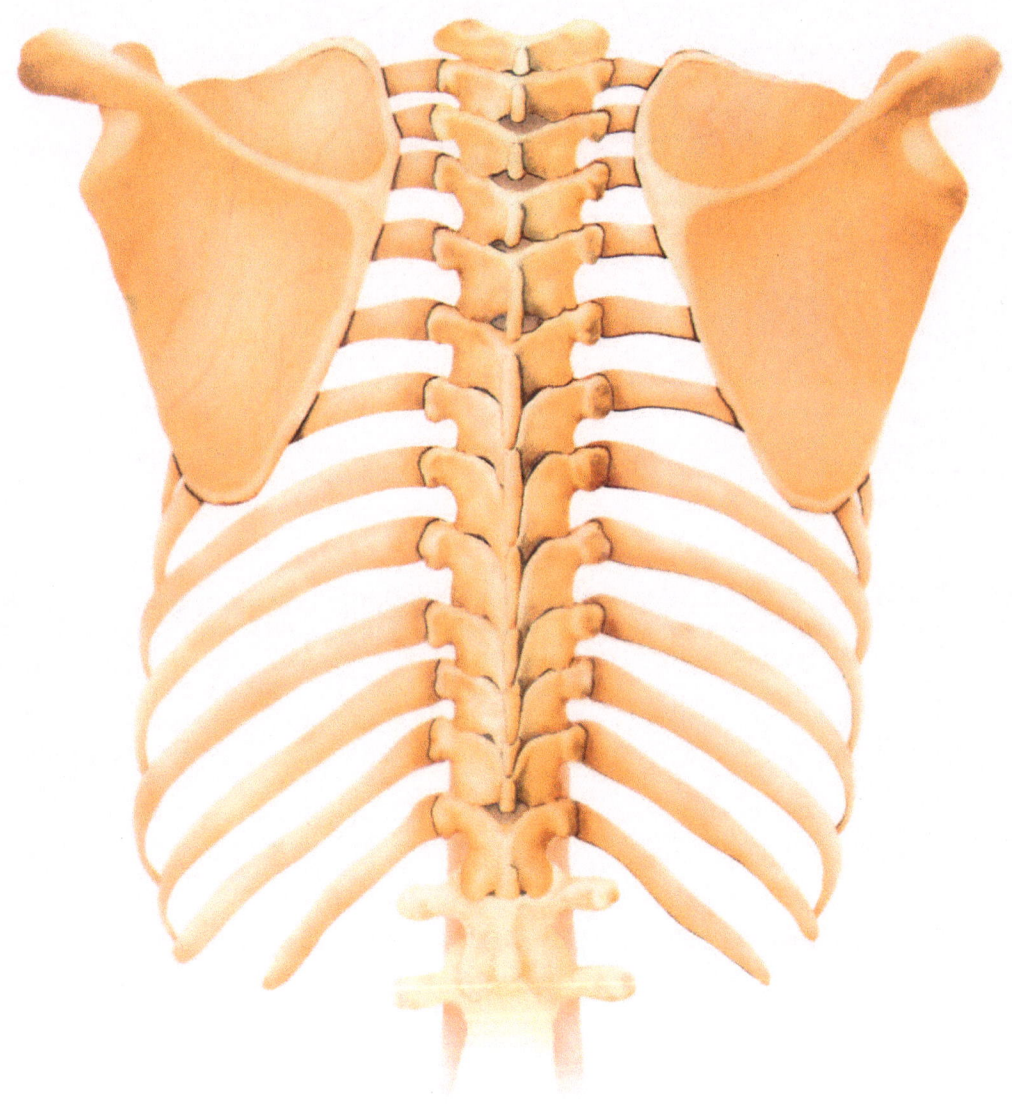

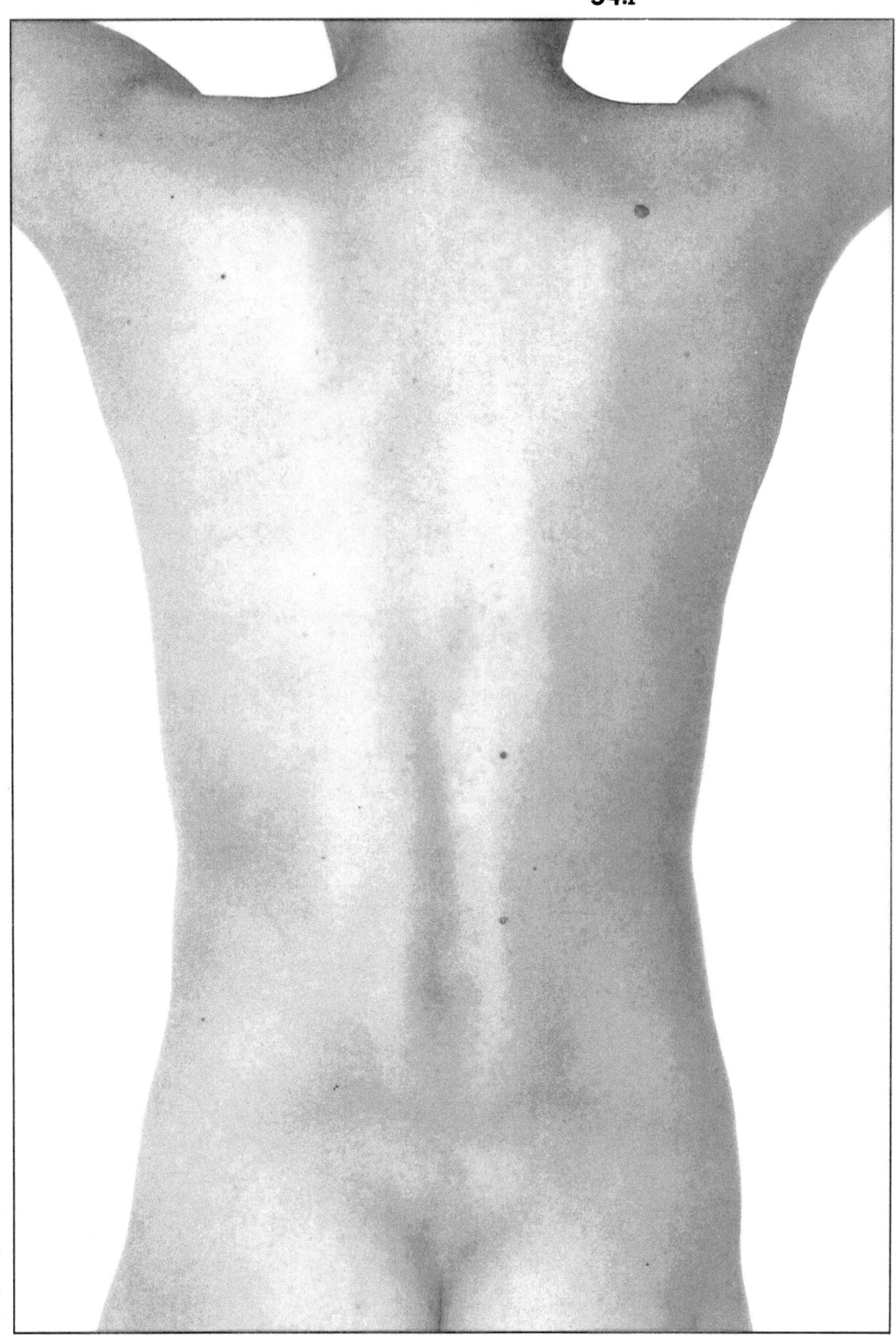

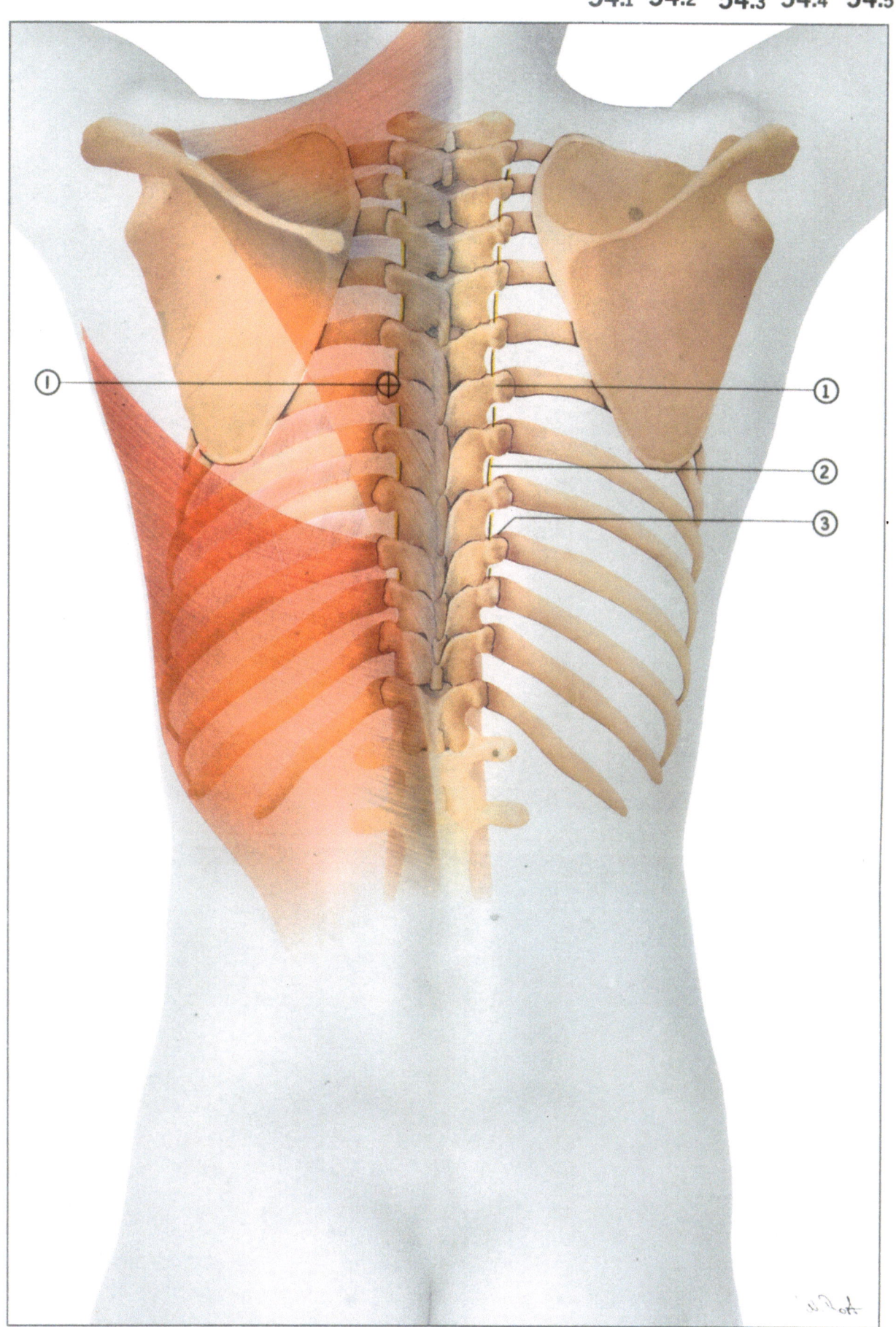

54

① Injection site for sympathetic block at T6. ① Transverse process of T6. ② Sympathetic trunk. ③ Head of 9th rib

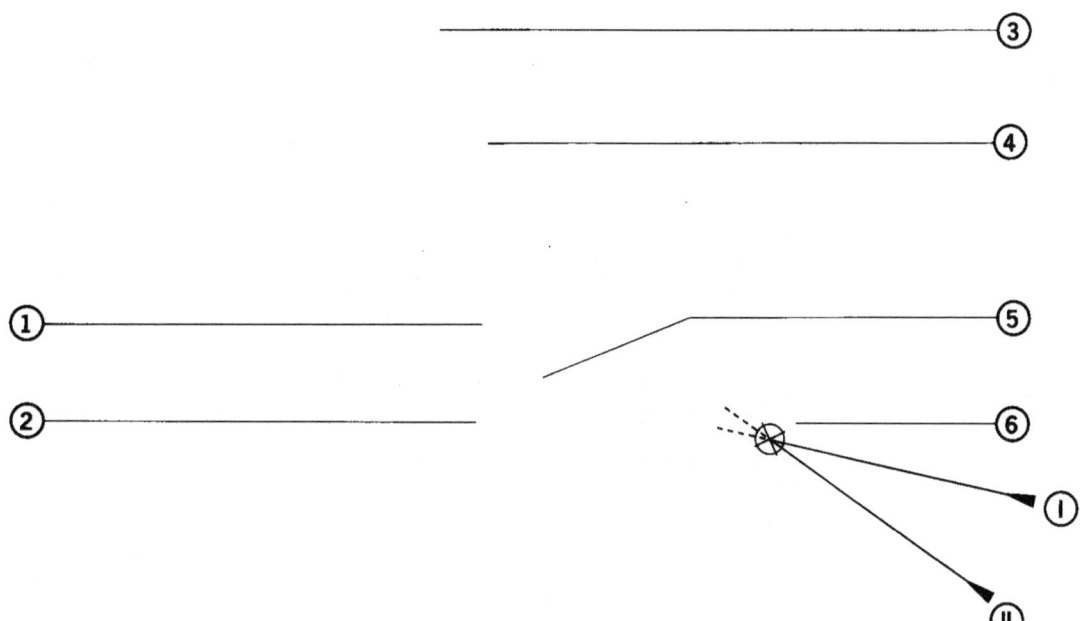

Ⓘ Injection site for celiac plexus block. Ⓘ Injection site for splanchnic nerve block. ① Body of T12. ② Body of L1. ③ Thoracic sympathetic trunk. ④ Greater splanchnic nerve. ⑤ Celiac plexus. ⑥ Twelfth rib

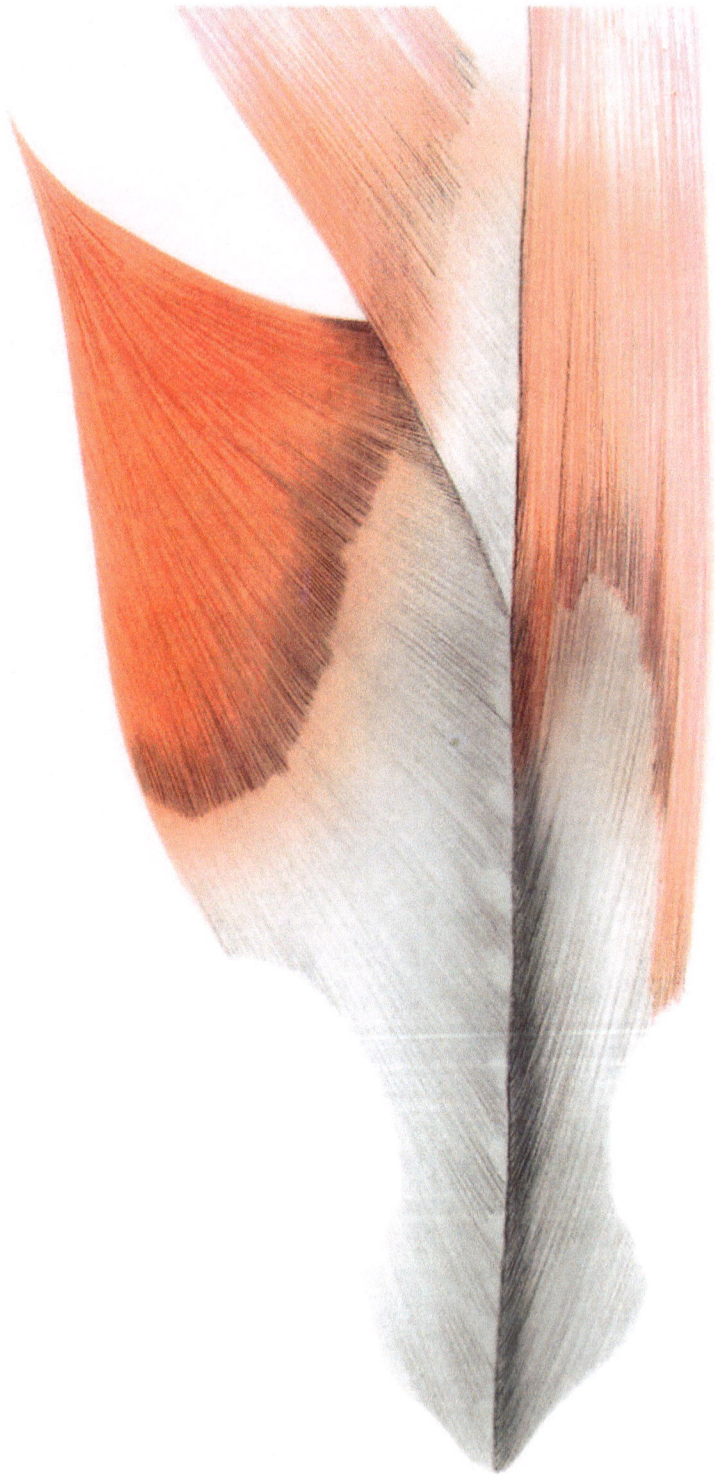

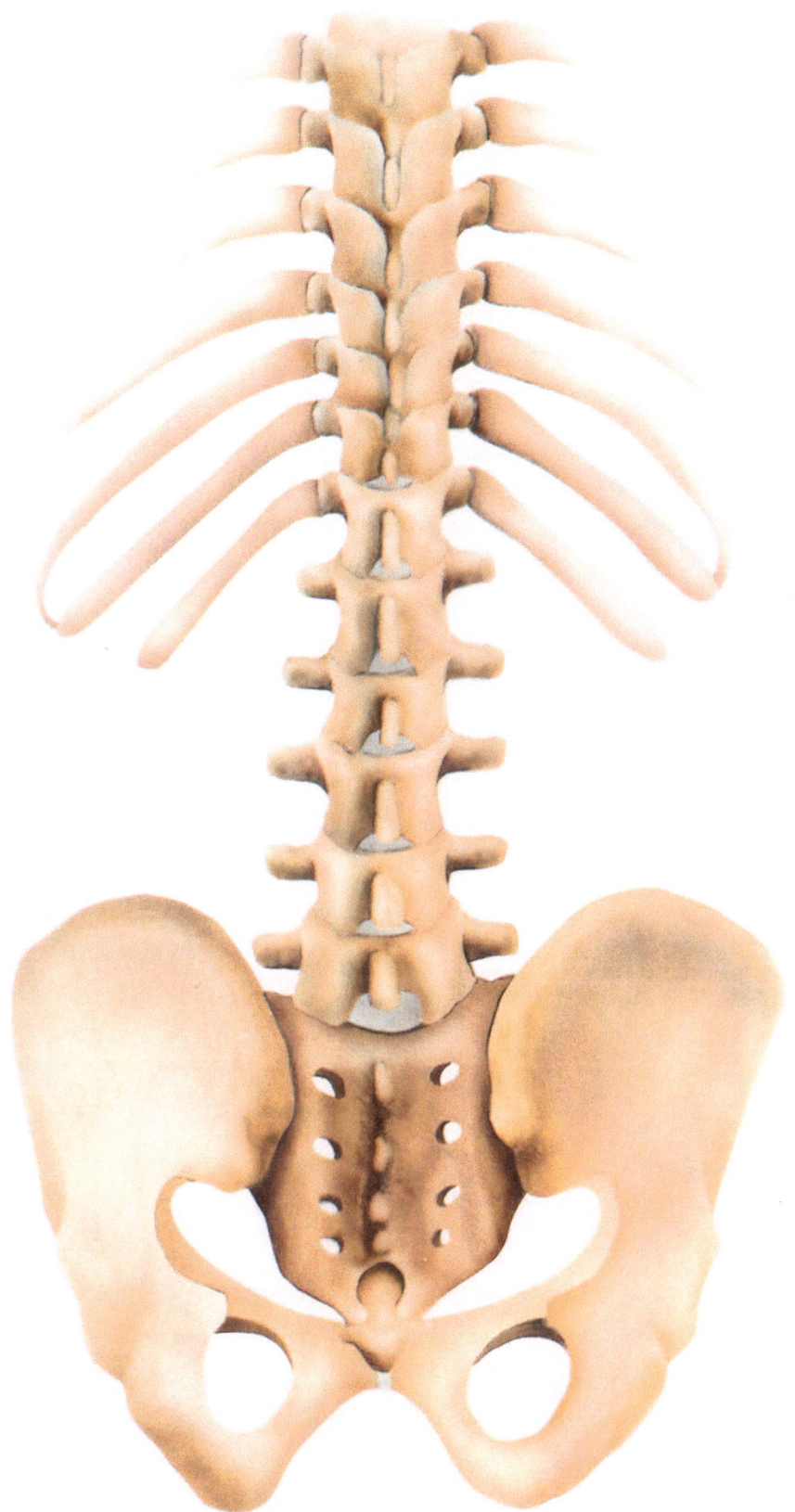

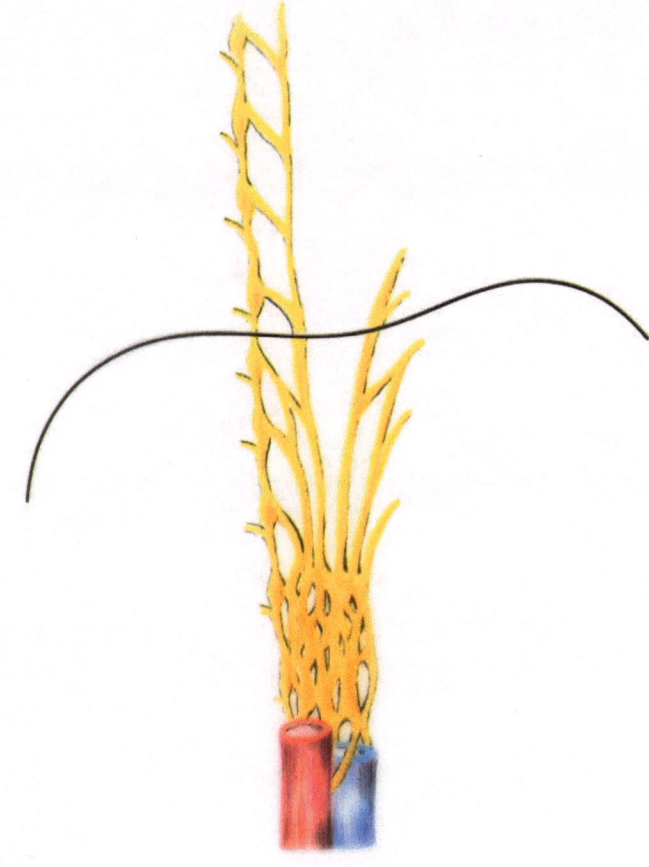

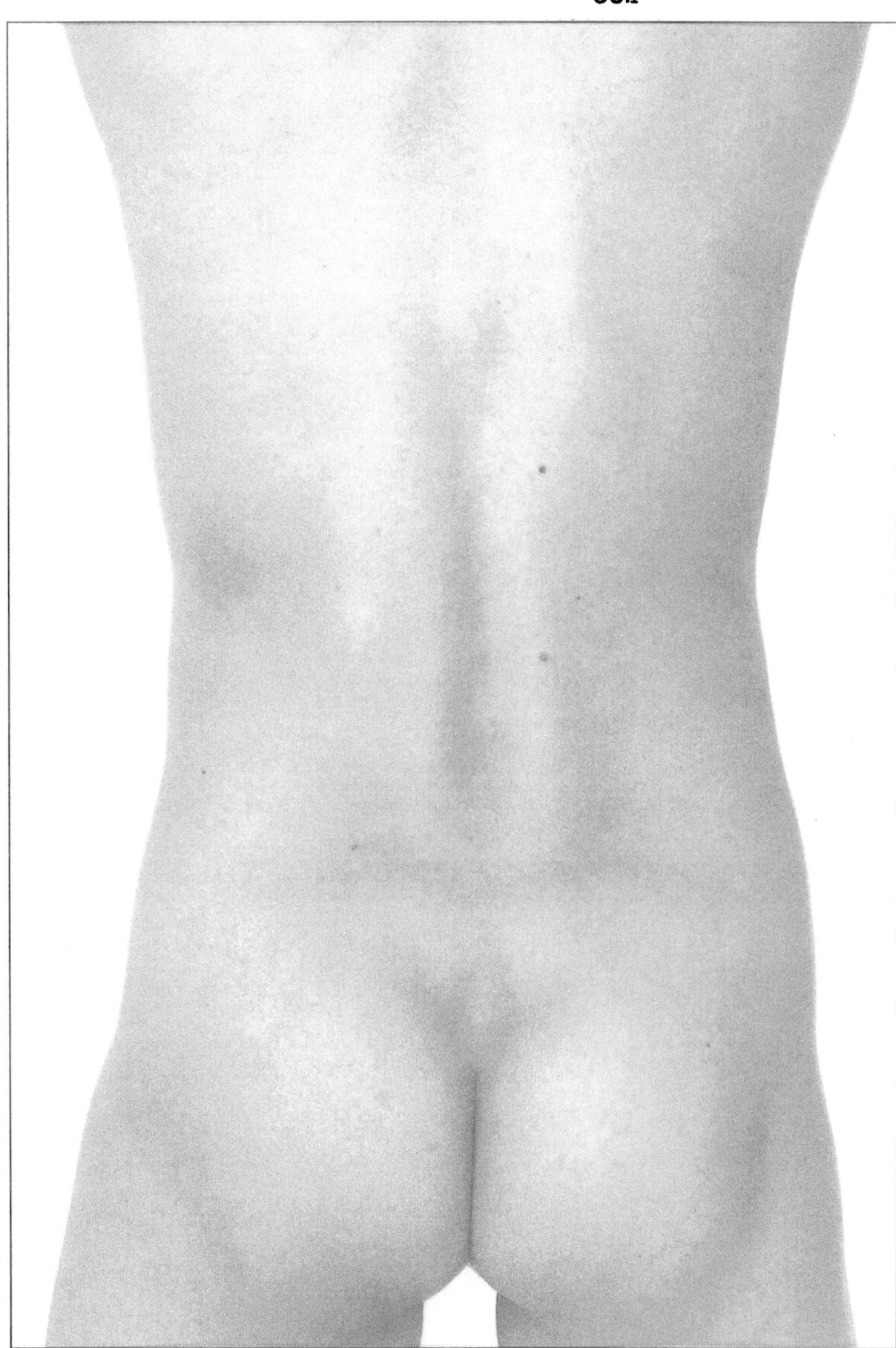

Splanchnic Nerve and Celiac Plexus Block

Splanchnic Nerve and Celiac Plexus Block

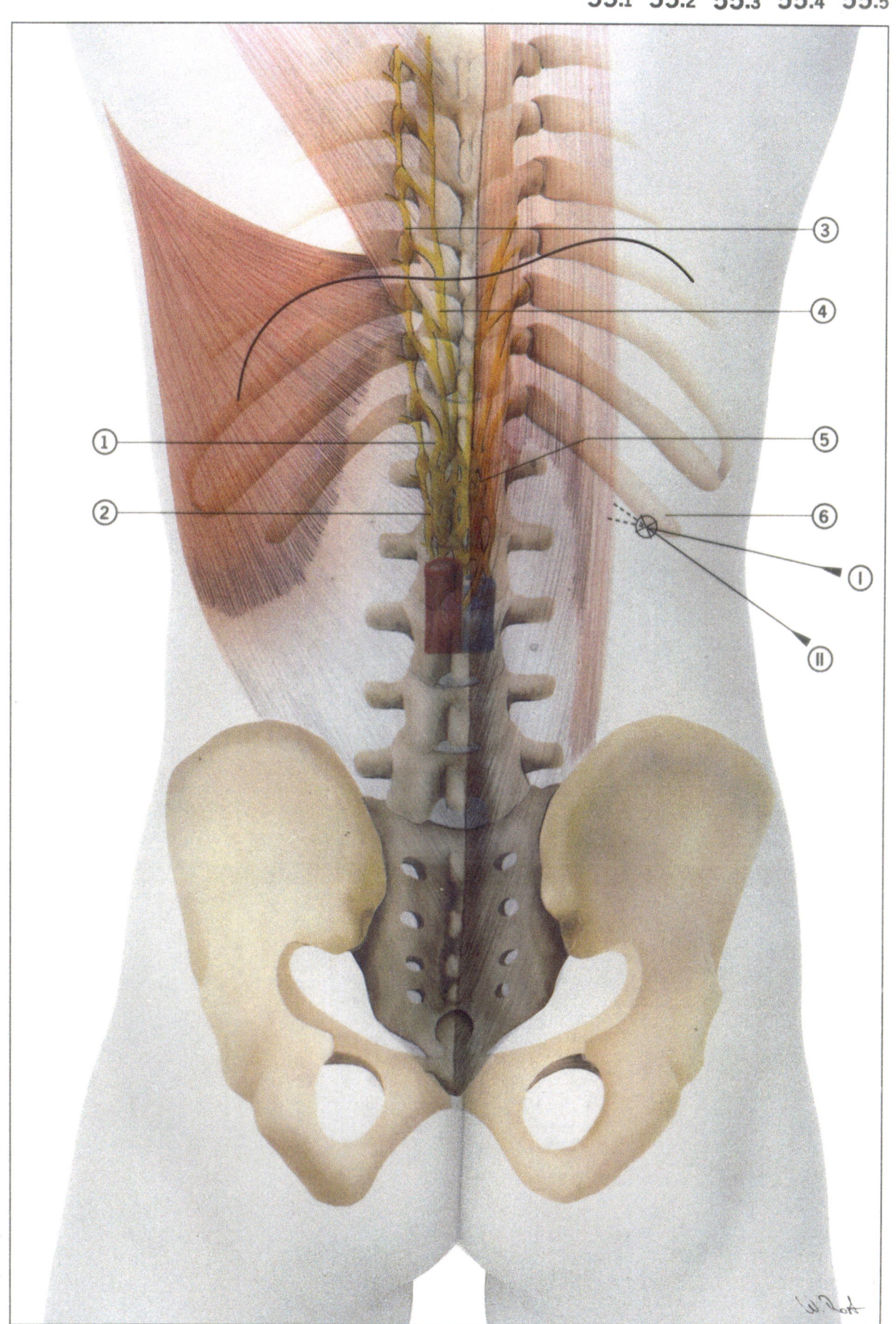

Ⅰ Injection site for celiac plexus block. Ⅱ Injection site for splanchnic nerve block. ① Body of T12. ② Body of L1. ③ Thoracic sympathetic trunk. ④ Greater splanchnic nerve. ⑤ Celiac plexus. ⑥ Twelfth rib

① ————————— ④
⊕
————————— ⑤
⊕

⊕

① ——————————
② ——————————
③ ——————————

① Injection sites overlying transverse processes of L2, L3, and L4. ① Transverse process of L2. ② Transverse process of L3. ③ Transverse process of L4. ④ Junction of lateral margin of erector spinae muscle and 12th rib. ⑤ Erector spinae muscle.

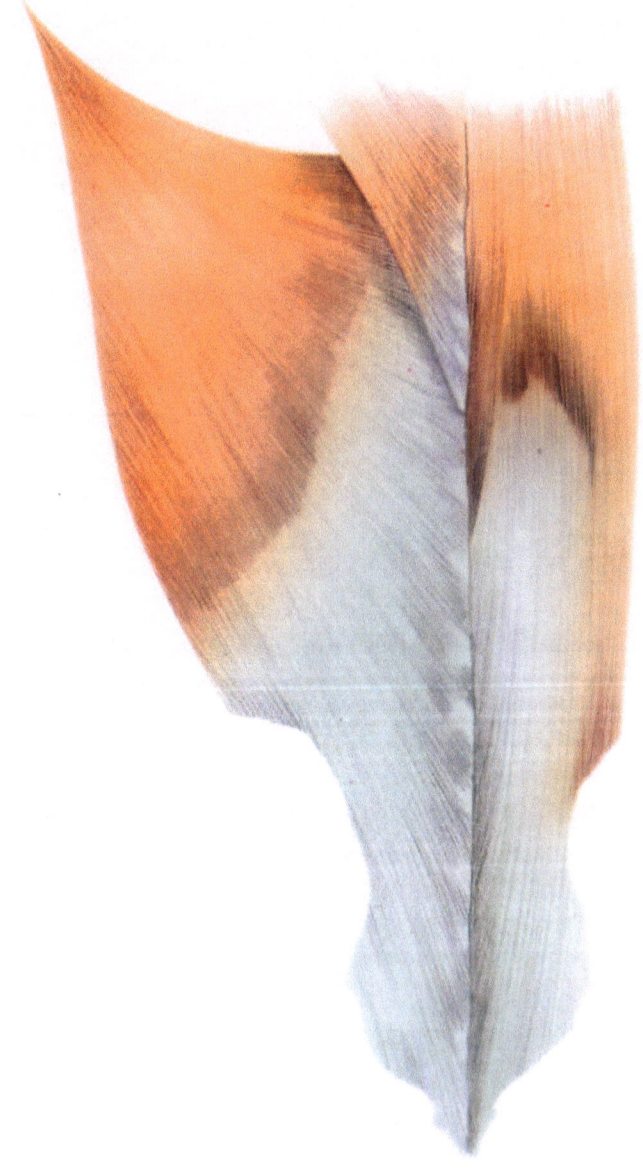

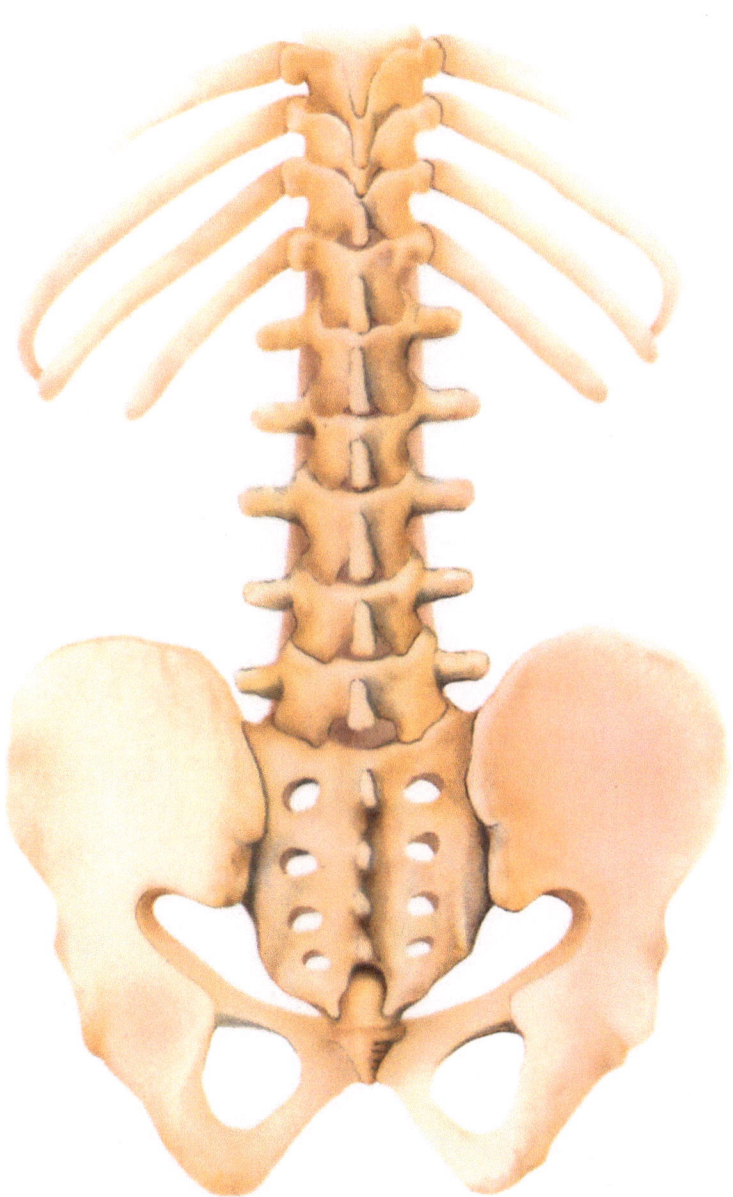

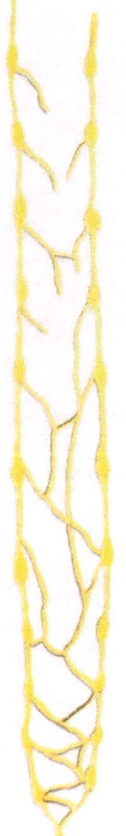

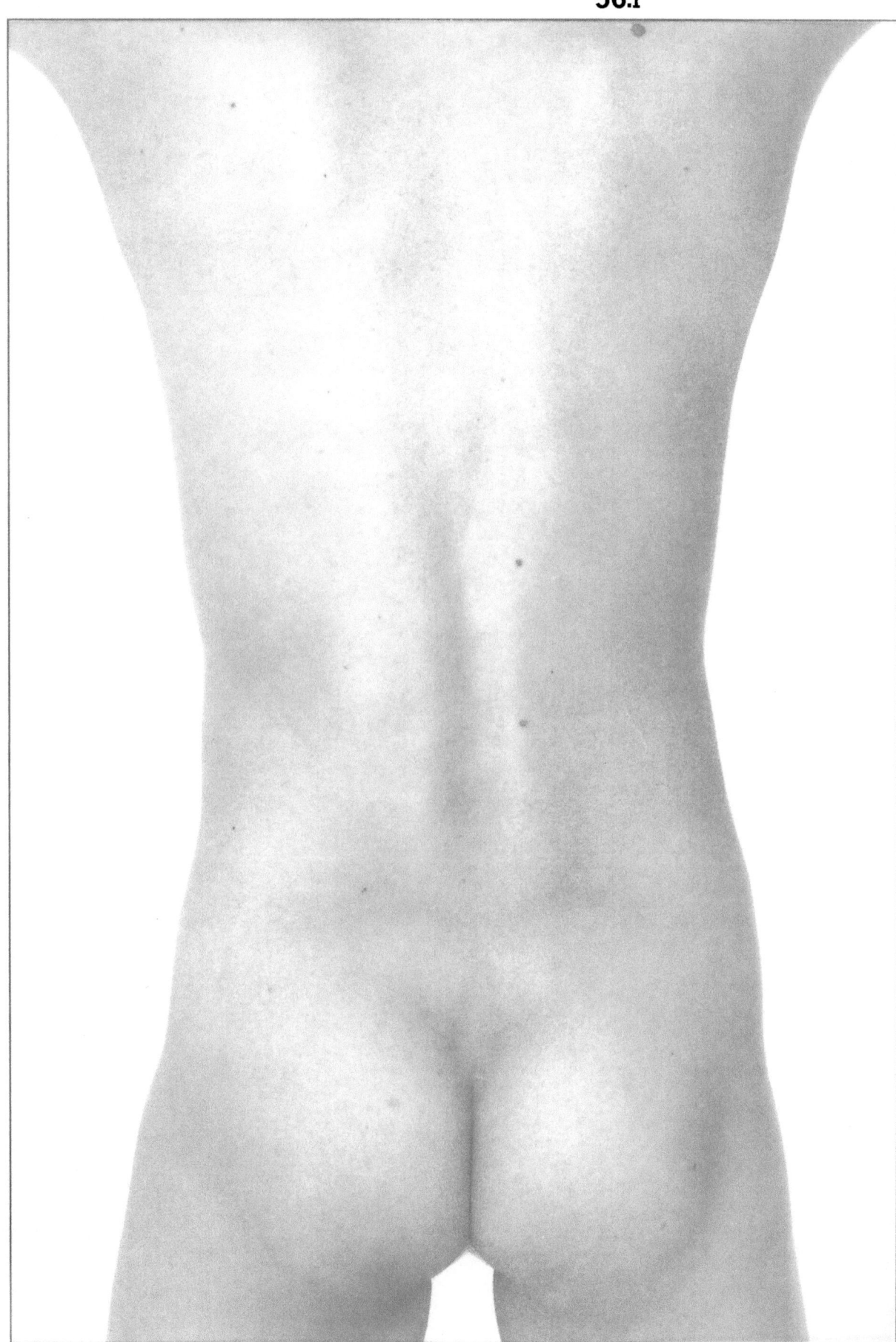

Lumbar Sympathetic Block: Paramedian Approach

Lumbar Sympathetic Block: Paramedian Approach

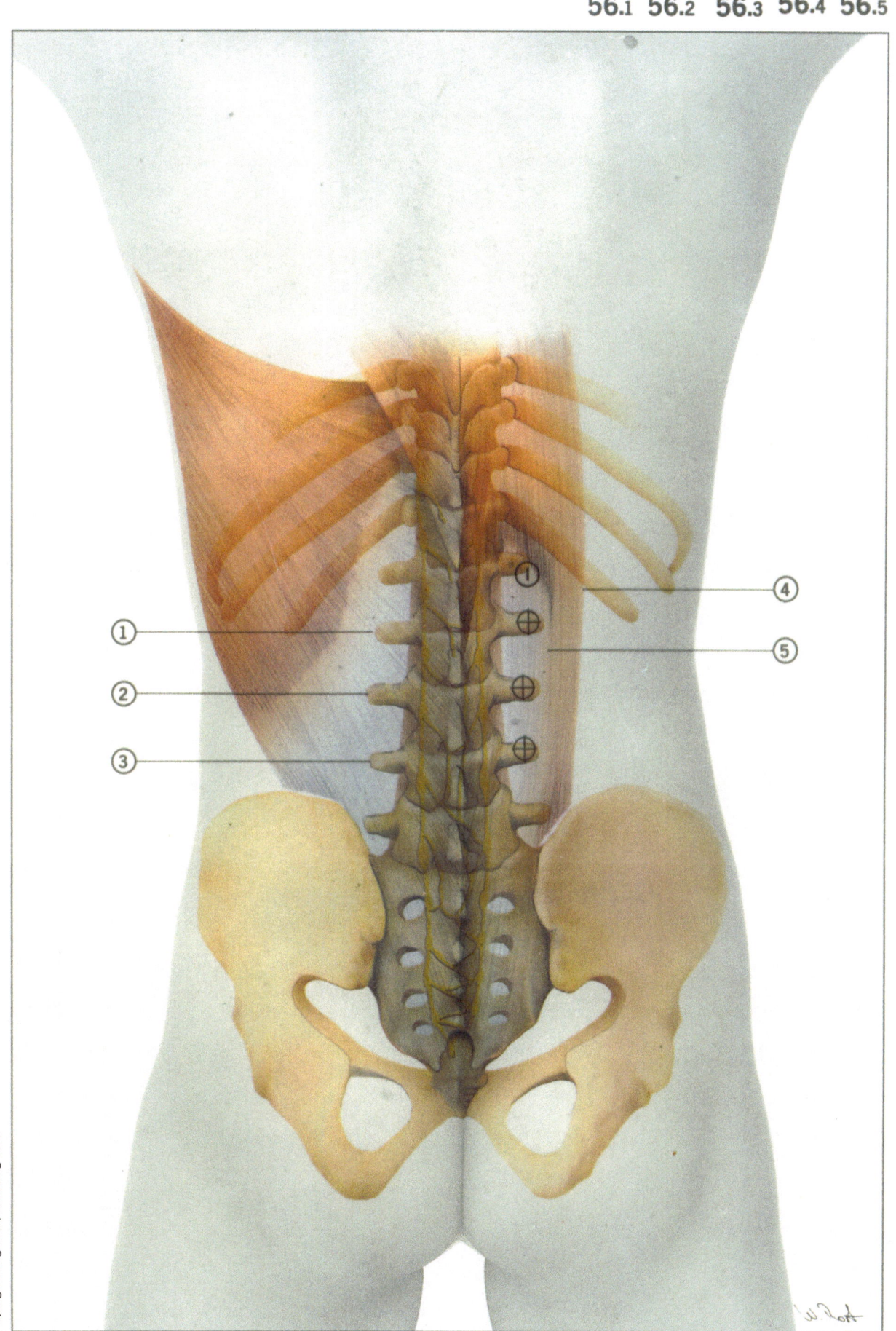

56

① Injection sites overlying transverse processes of L2, L3, and L4. ① Transverse process of L2. ② Transverse process of L3. ③ Transverse process of L4. ④ Junction of lateral margin of erector spinae muscle and 12th rib. ⑤ Erector spinae muscle.

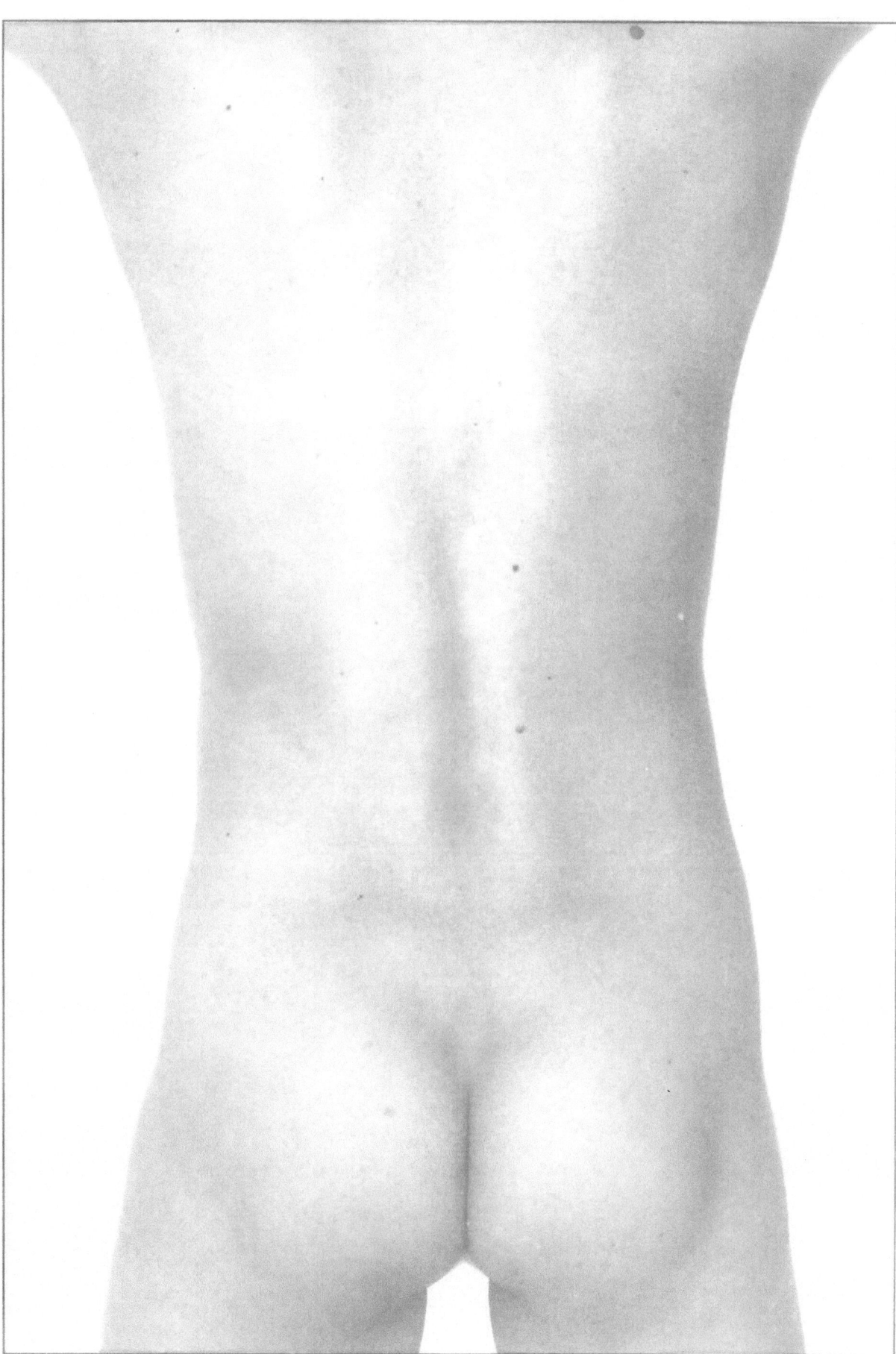

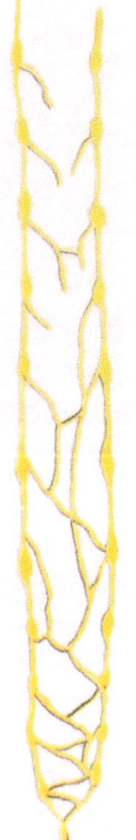

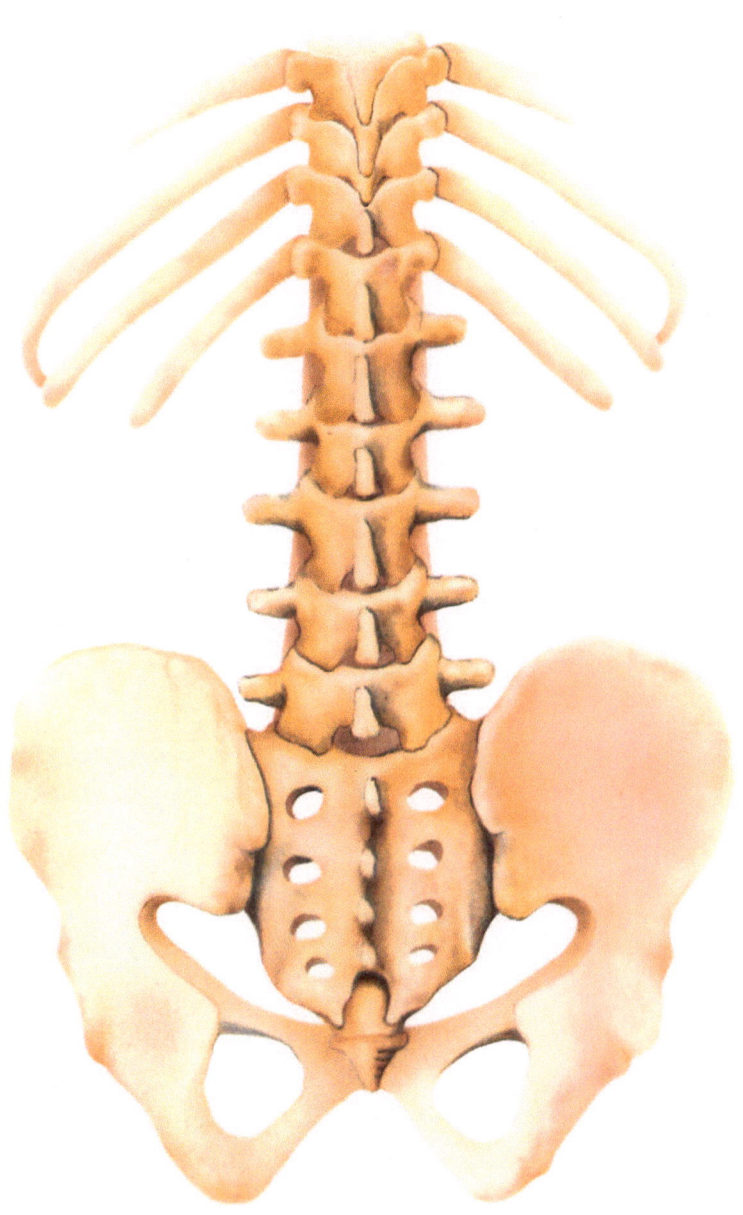

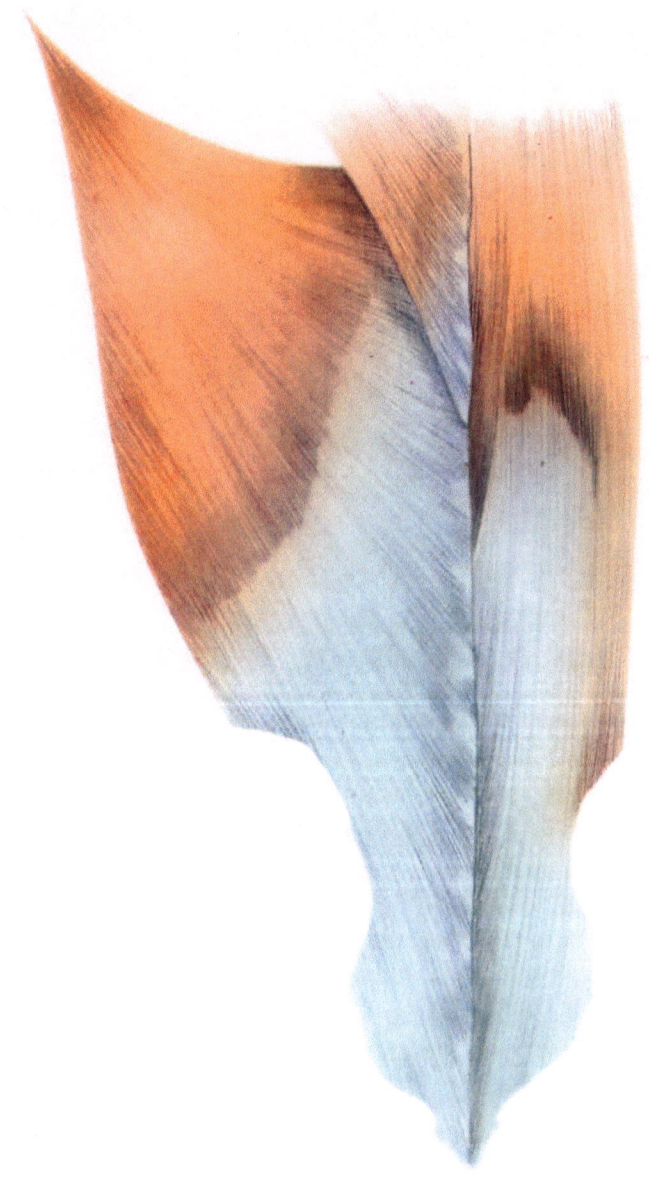

© Springer-Verlag Berlin, Heidelberg 1988

① Injection sites for lateral (Reid's) approach in lumbar sympathetic block. ① Junction of lateral margin of erector spinae muscle and 12th rib. ② Transverse process of L2. ③ Transverse process of L3. ④ Transverse process of L4

Lumbar Sympathetic Block: Lateral Approach

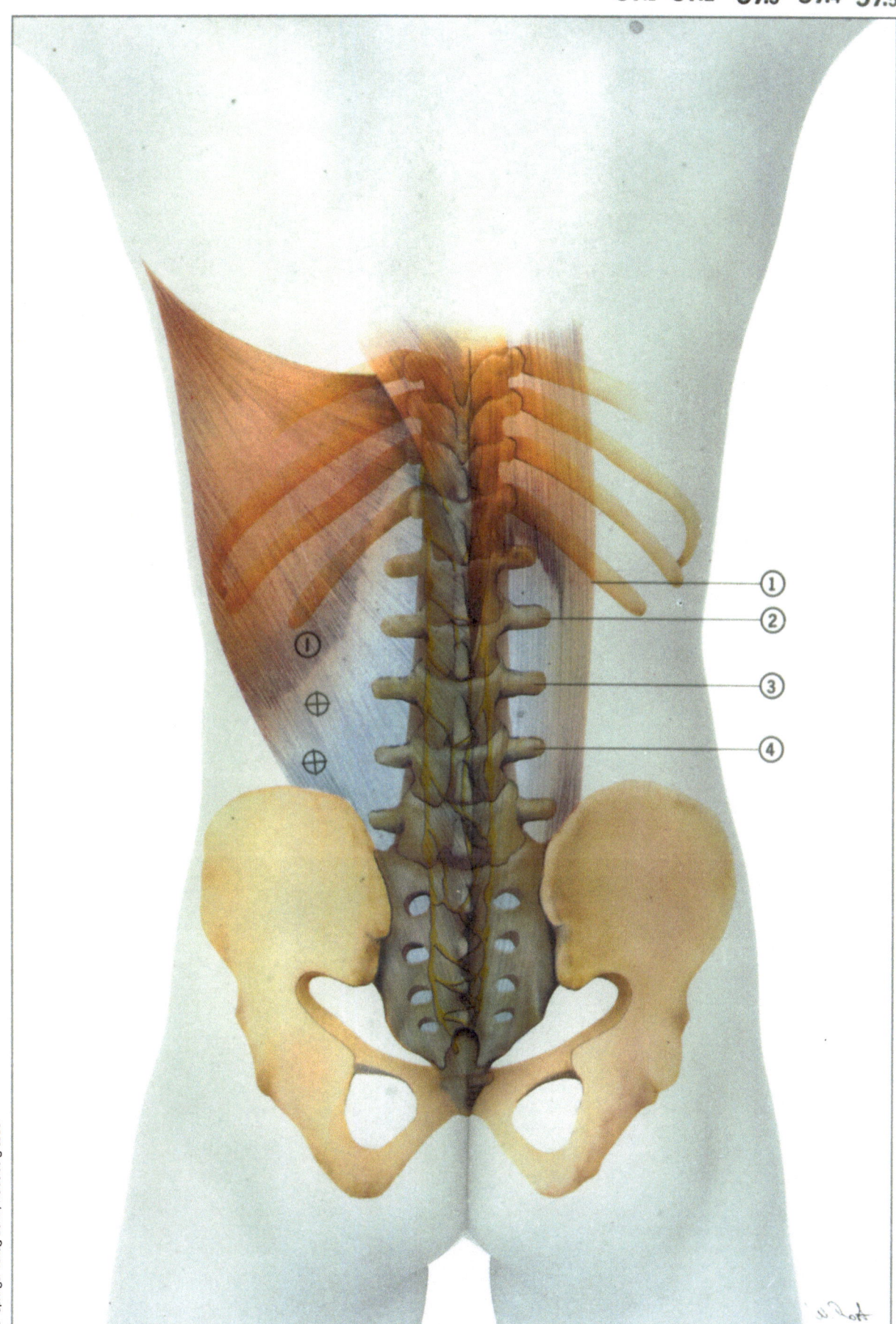

57

① Injection sites for lateral (Reid's) approach in lumbar sympathetic block. ① Junction of lateral margin of erector spinae muscle and 12th rib.
② Transverse process of L2. ③ Transverse process of L3. ④ Transverse process of L4

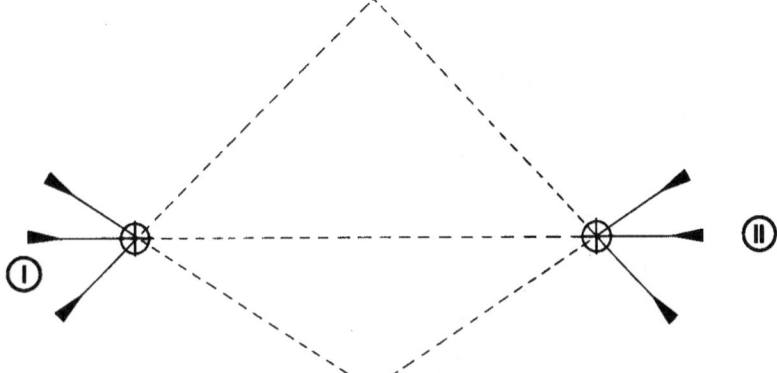

① Injection site at the equator of the breast (approximately at 4th rib). ② Injection site at sternocostal junction

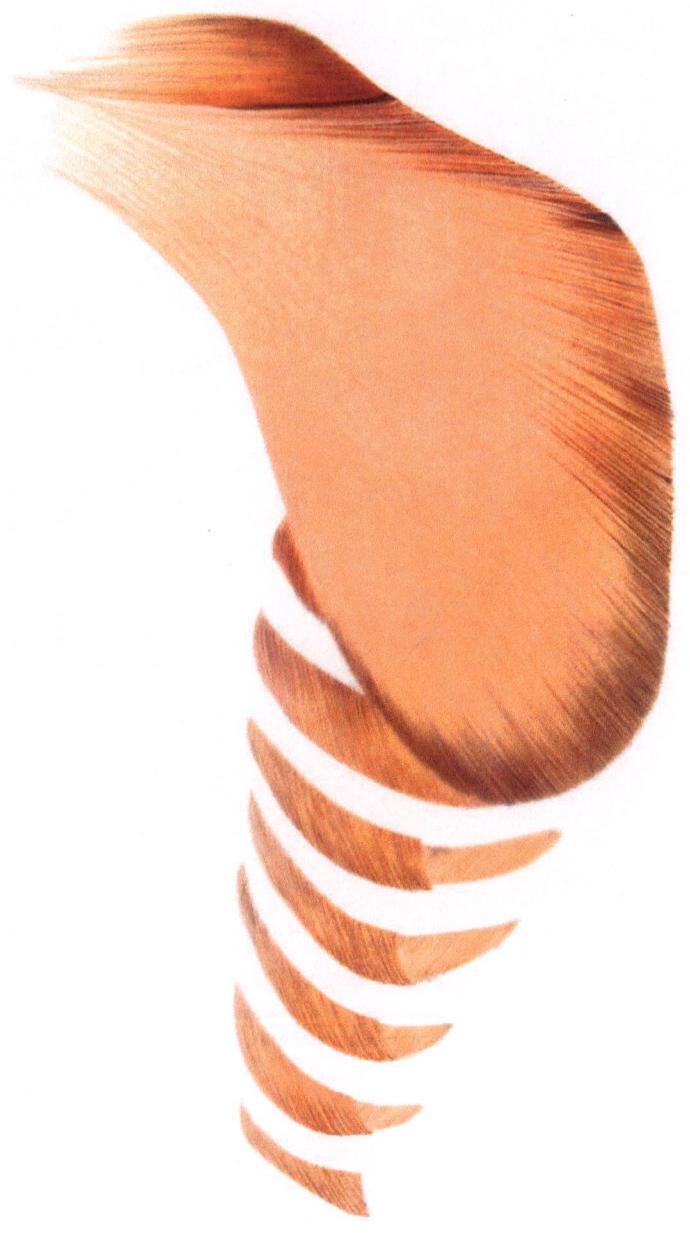

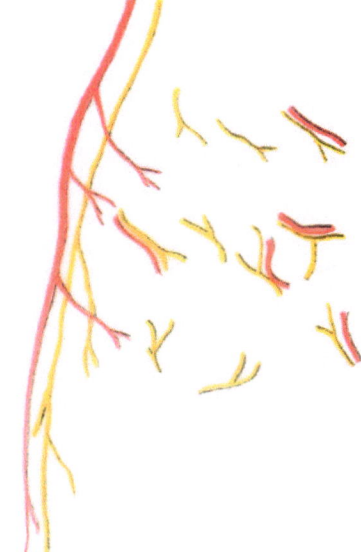

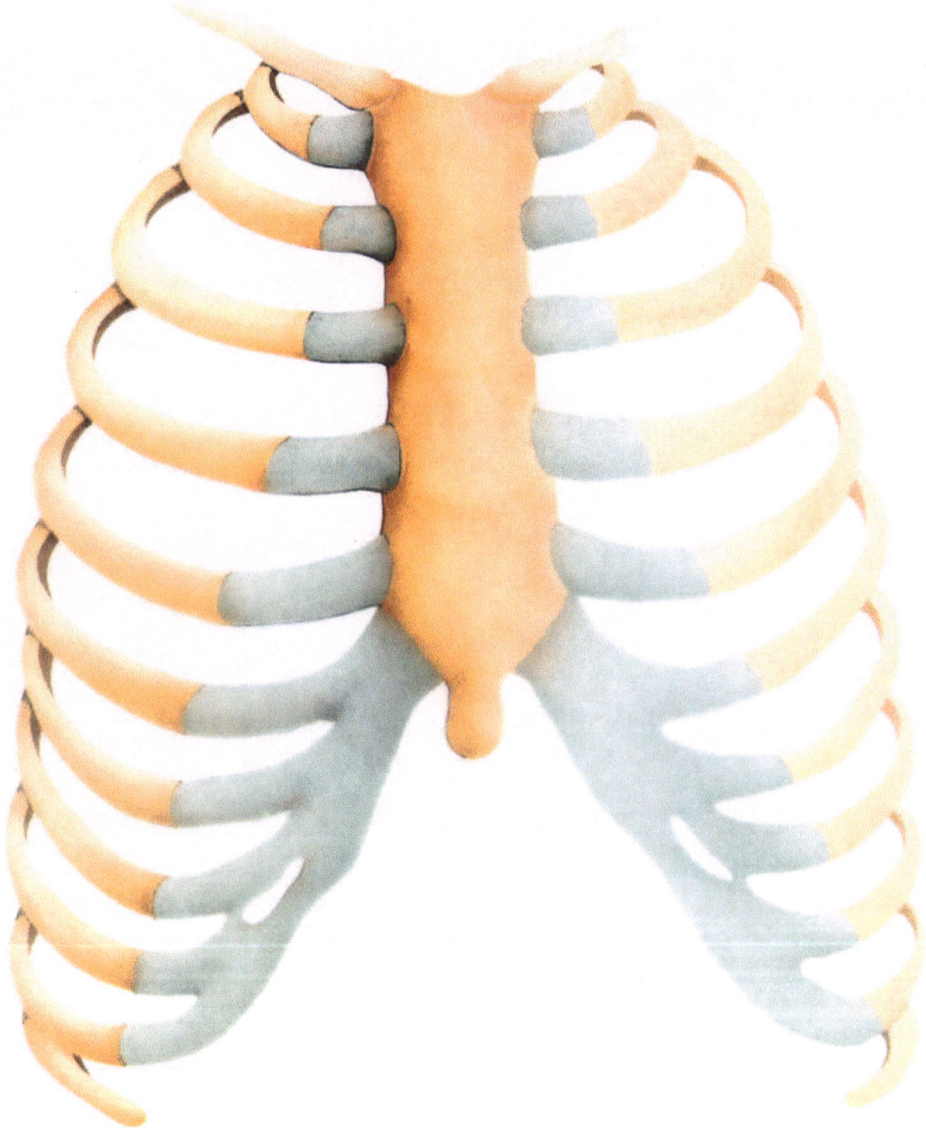

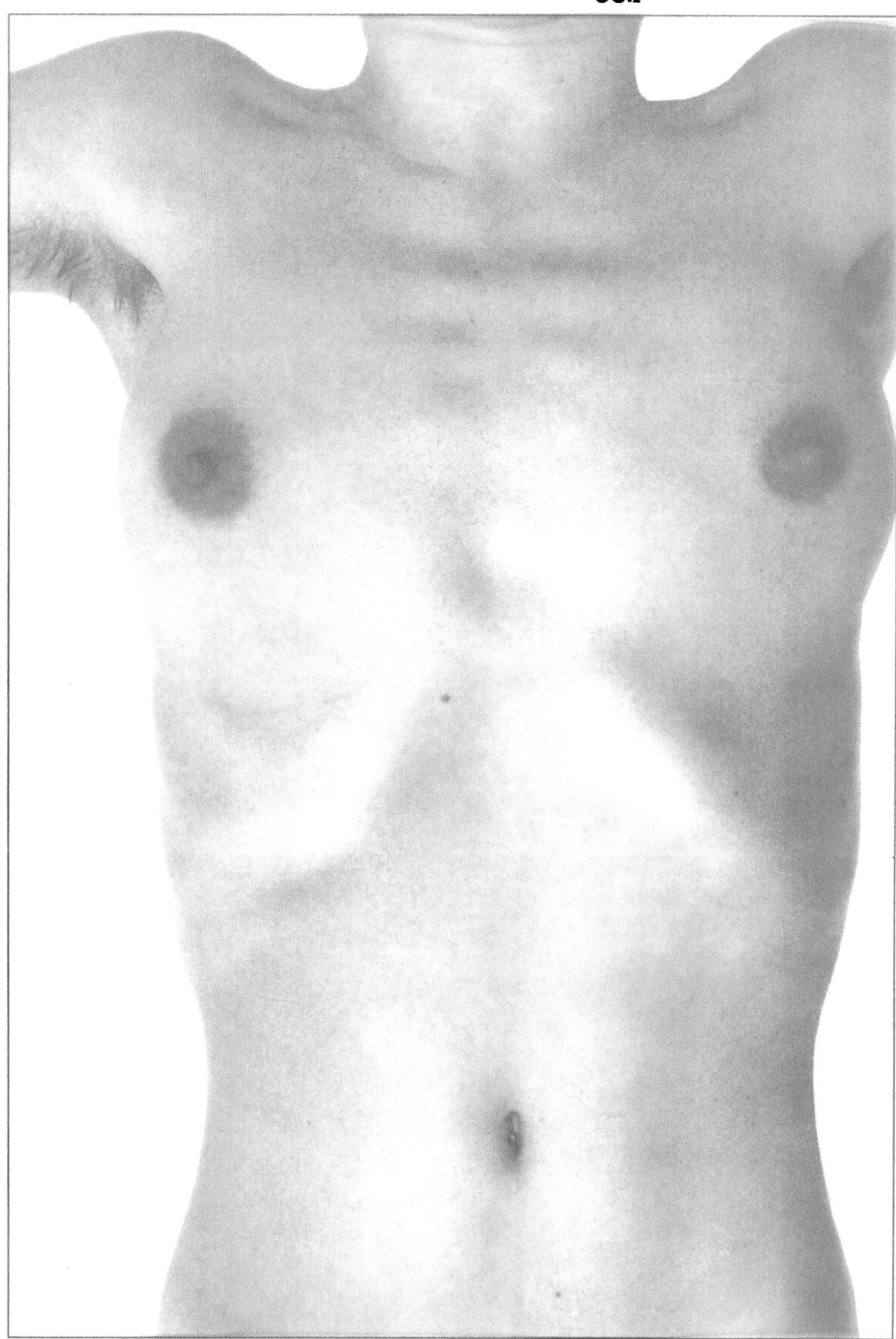

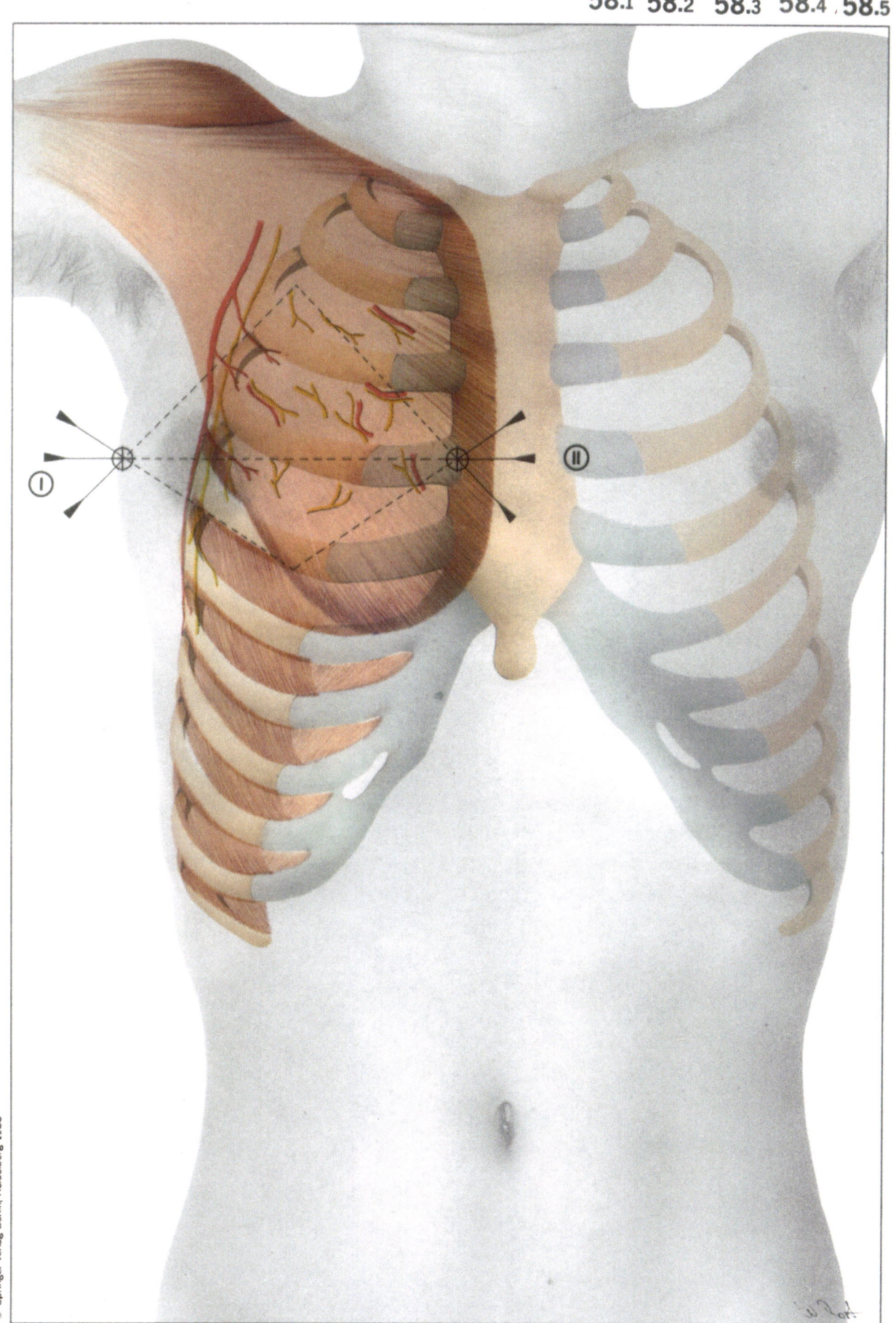

① Injection site at the equator of the breast (approximately at 4th rib). ② Injection site at sternocostal junction

Infiltration for upper and lower laparotomy. ⊕ Points of needle entry. ✕ Subfascial depots along the linea alba

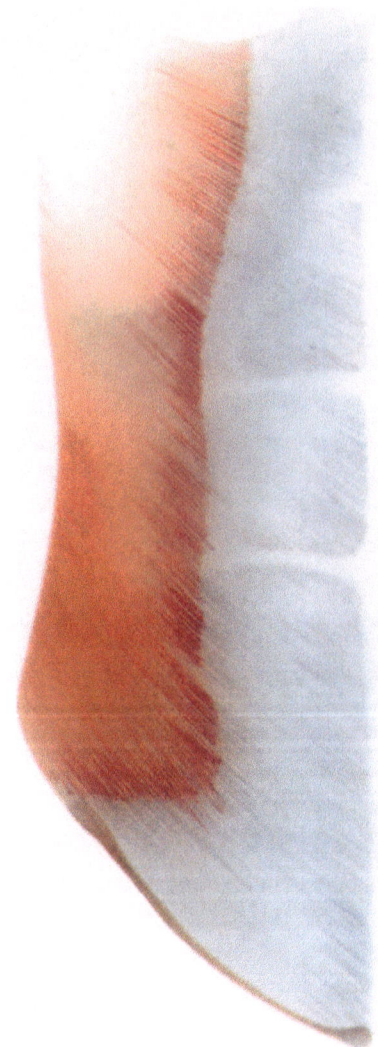

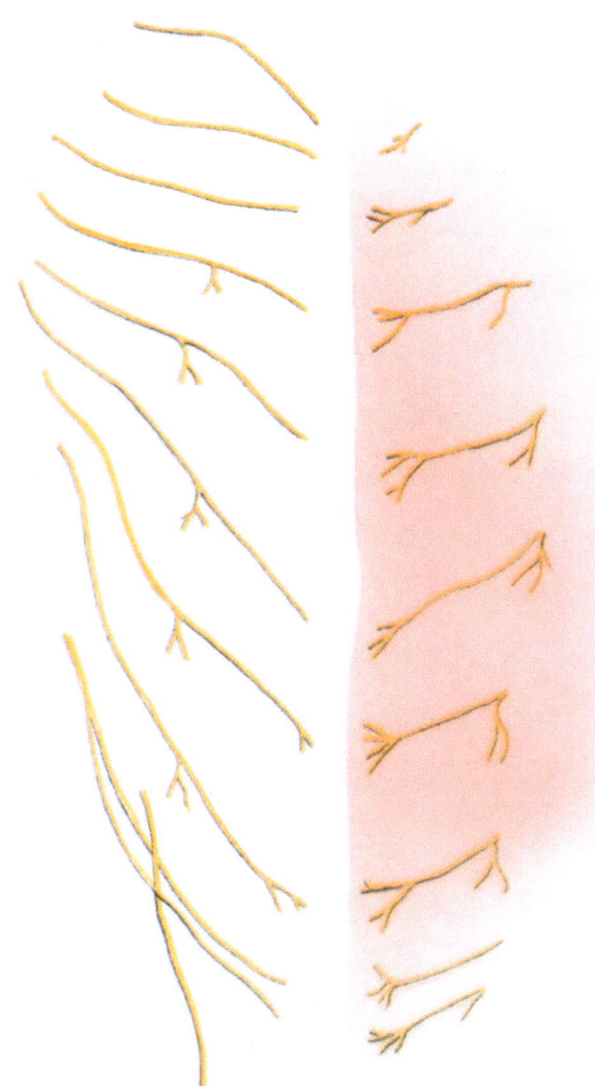

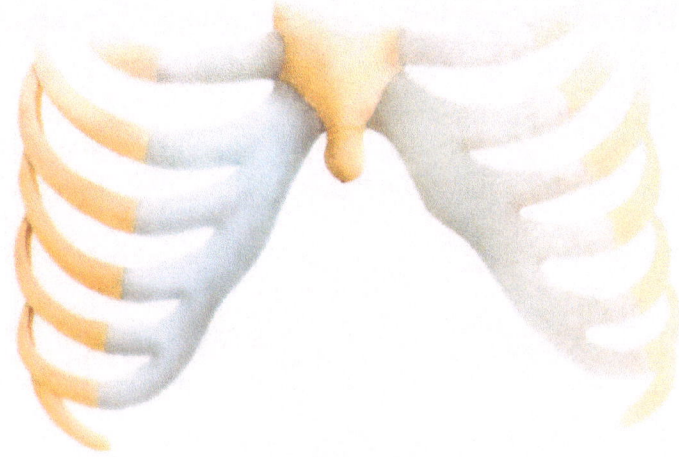

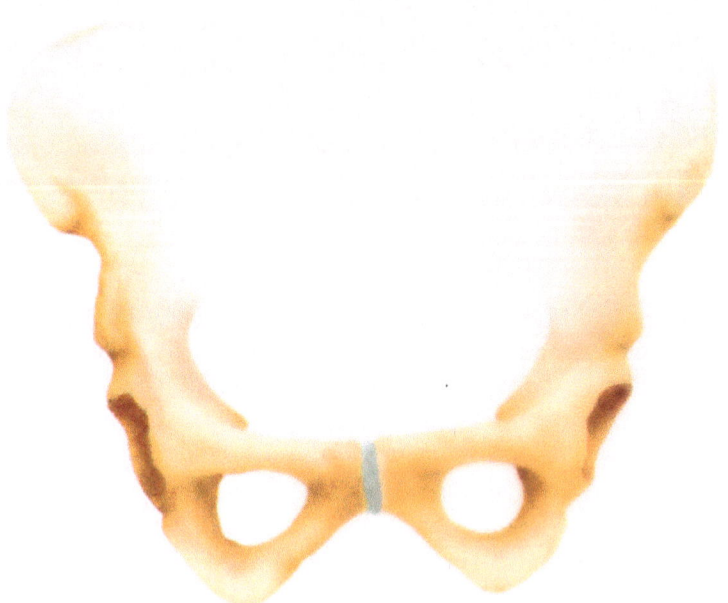

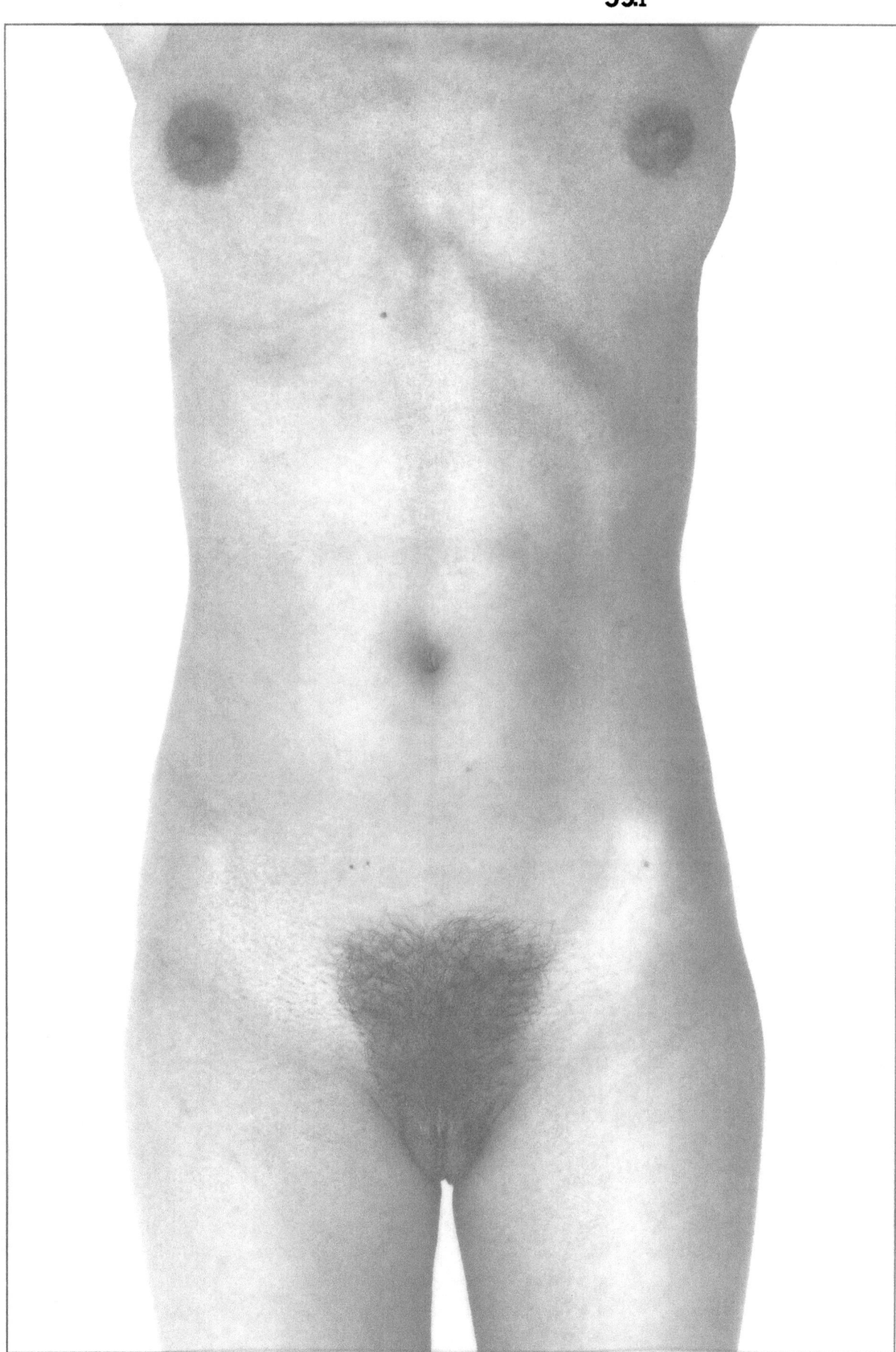

Field Block of Upper and Lower Abdomen

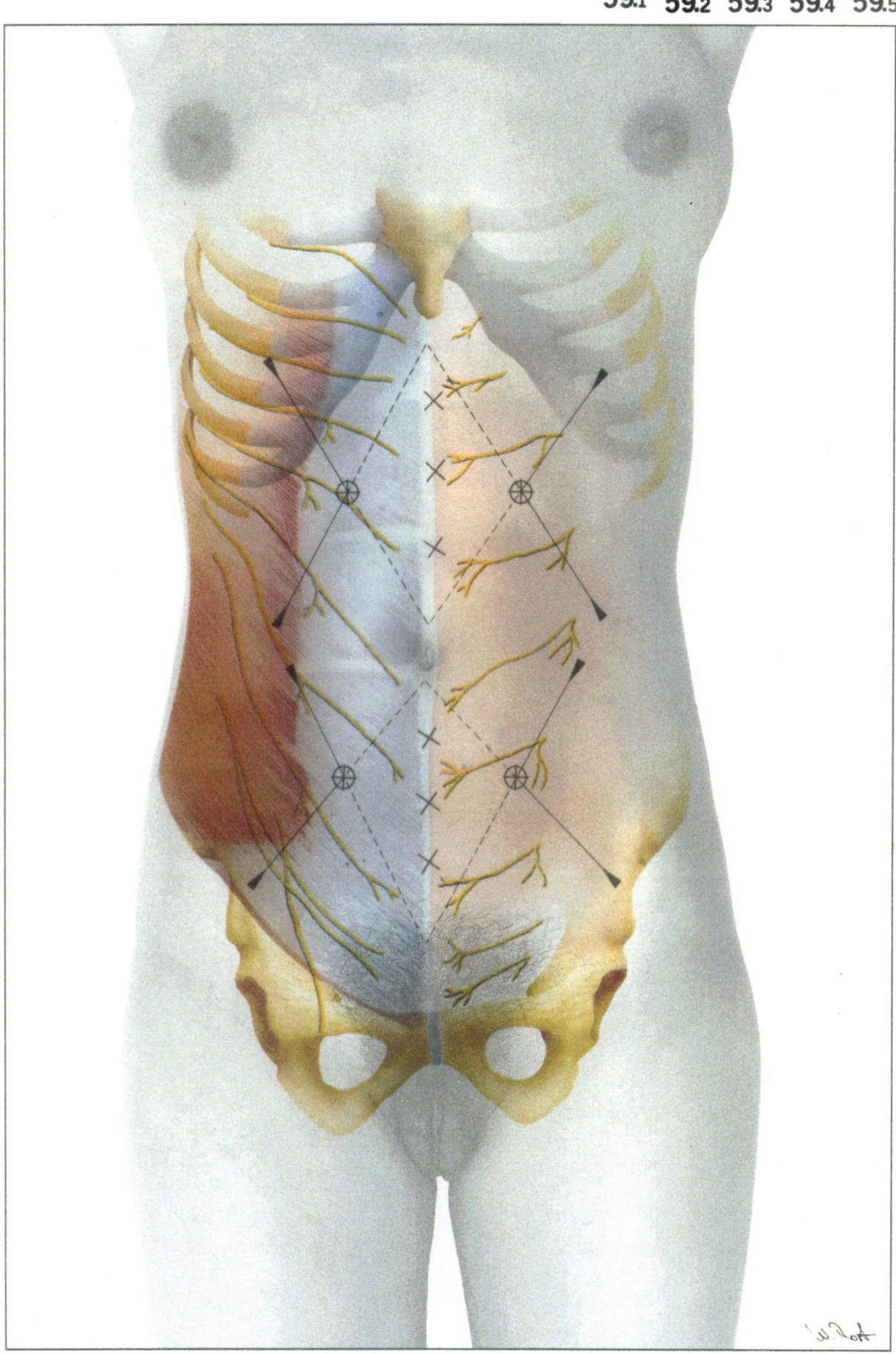

Infiltration for upper and lower laparotomy. ⊕ Points of needle entry. × Subfascial depots along the linea alba

① Injection site medial to anterior superior iliac spine. ② Injection site above pubic tubercle. ① Anterior superior iliac spine. ② Inguinal ligament. ③ Spermatic cord. ④ Femoral nerve. ⑤ Femoral artery. ⑥ Femoral vein. ⑦ Iliac crest. ⑧ Nerves supplying inguinal region (iliohypogastric and ilioinguinal nerves). ⑨ Pubis

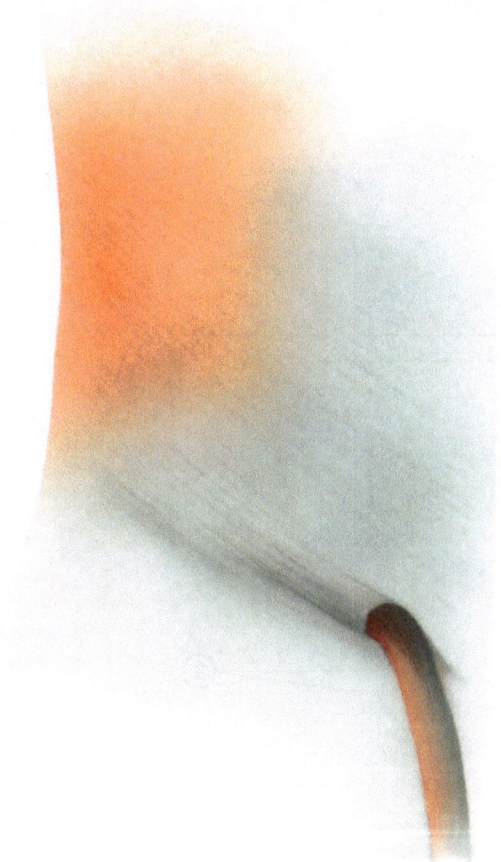

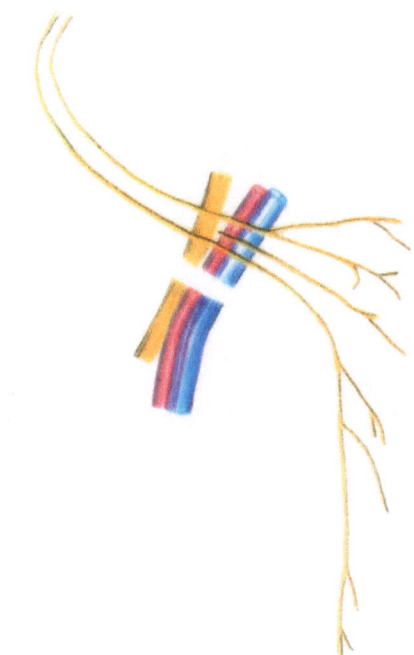

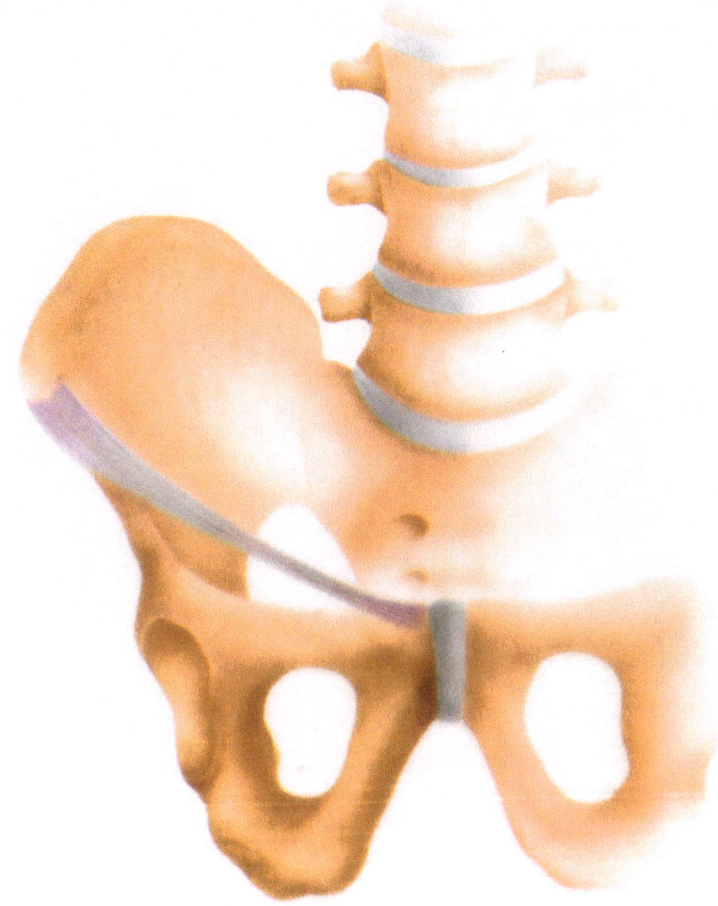

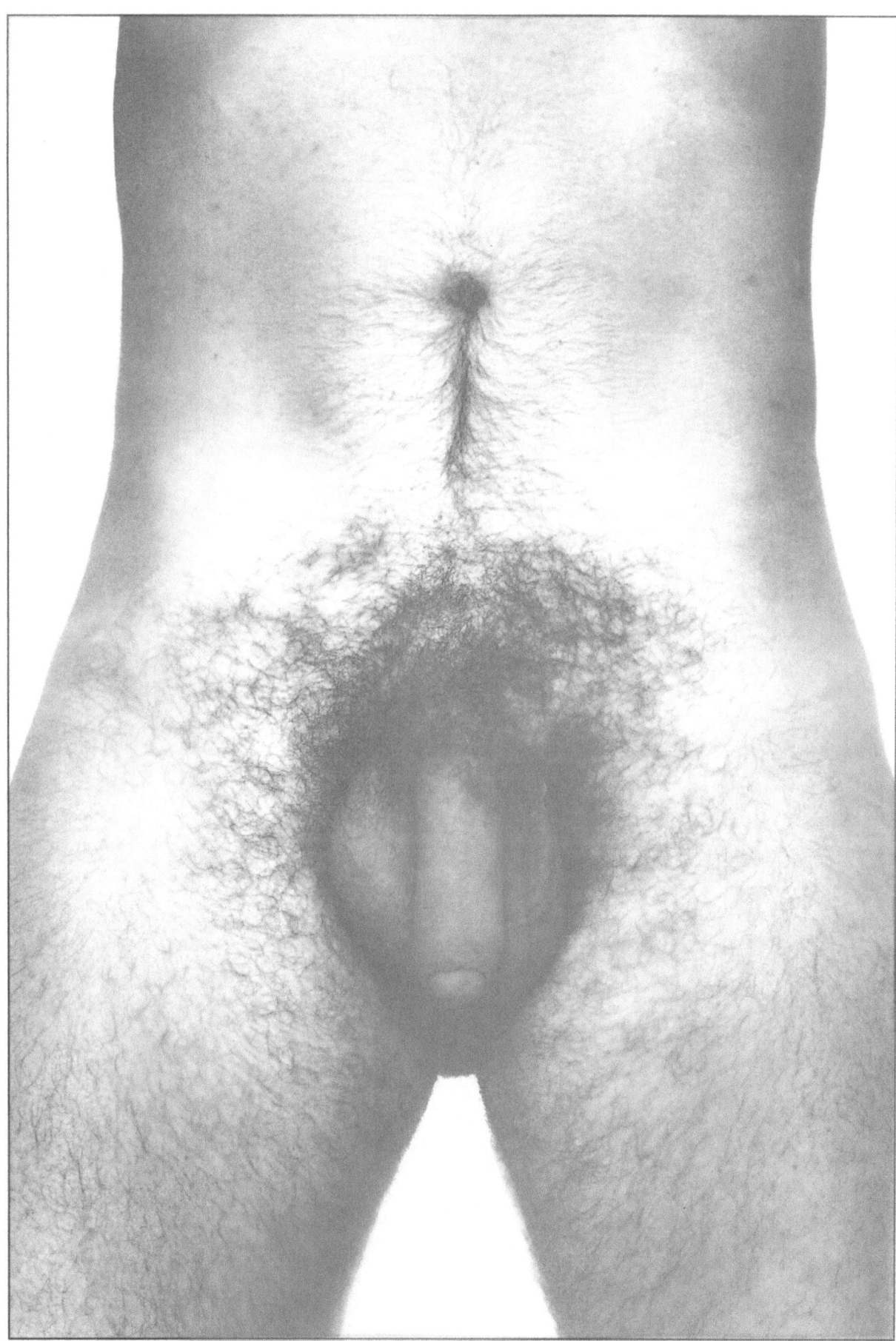

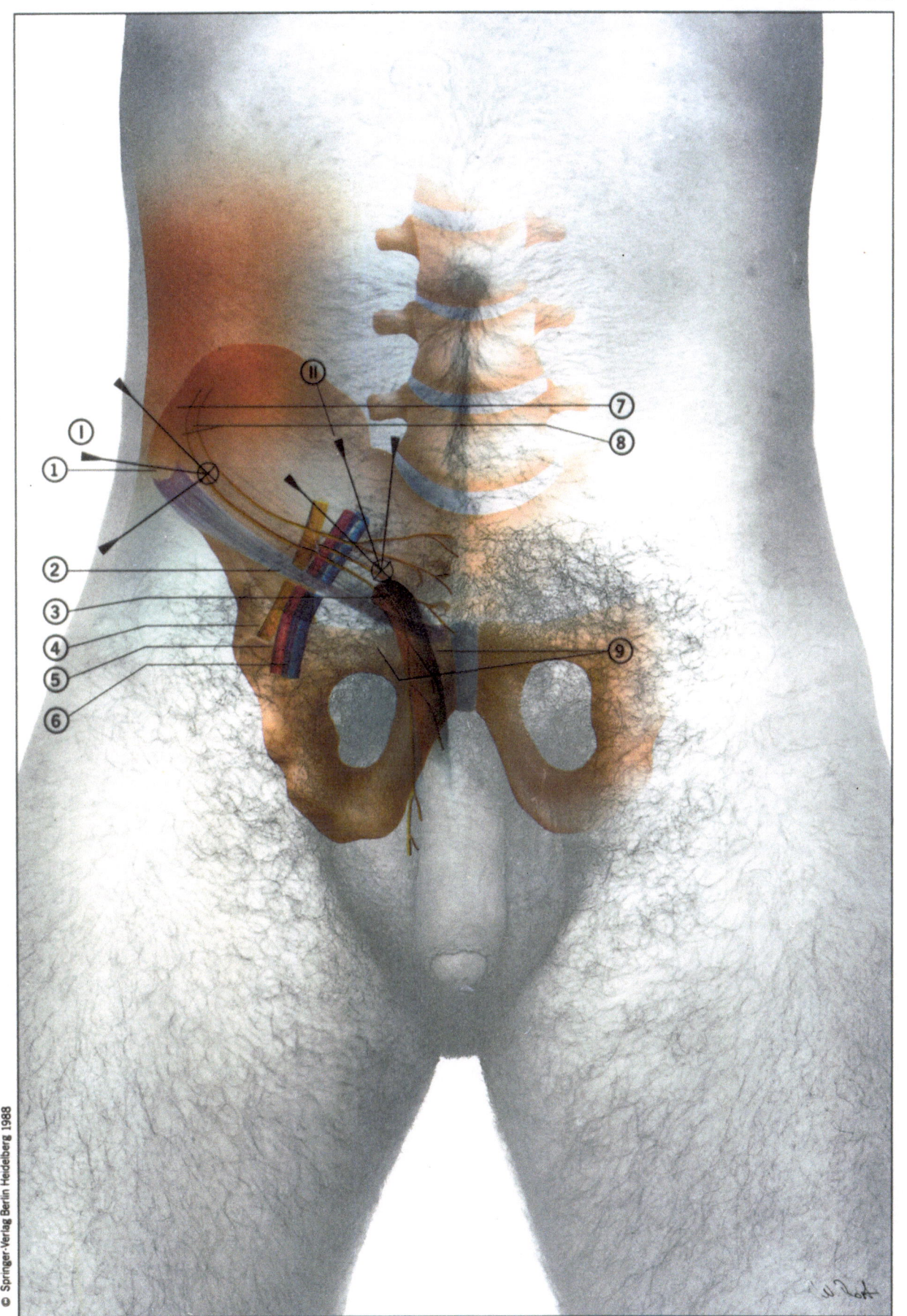

60

① Injection site medial to anterior superior iliac spine. ⑪ Injection site above pubic tubercle. ① Anterior superior iliac spine. ② Inguinal ligament. ③ Spermatic cord. ④ Femoral nerve. ⑤ Femoral artery. ⑥ Femoral vein. ⑦ Iliac crest. ⑧ Nerves supplying inguinal region (iliohypogastric and ilioinguinal nerves). ⑨ Pubis

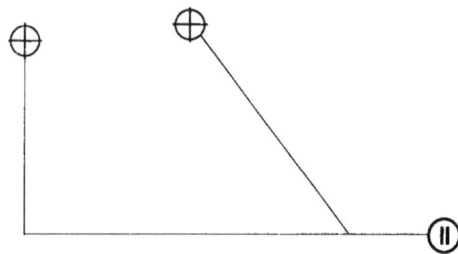

Ⓘ Points of entry for block at root of penis. Ⓘ Points of entry for block of prepuce. ① Dorsal penile artery. ② Dorsal penile vein. ③ Main nerve supply to penis

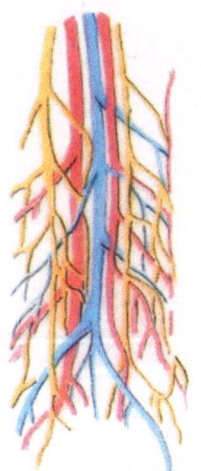

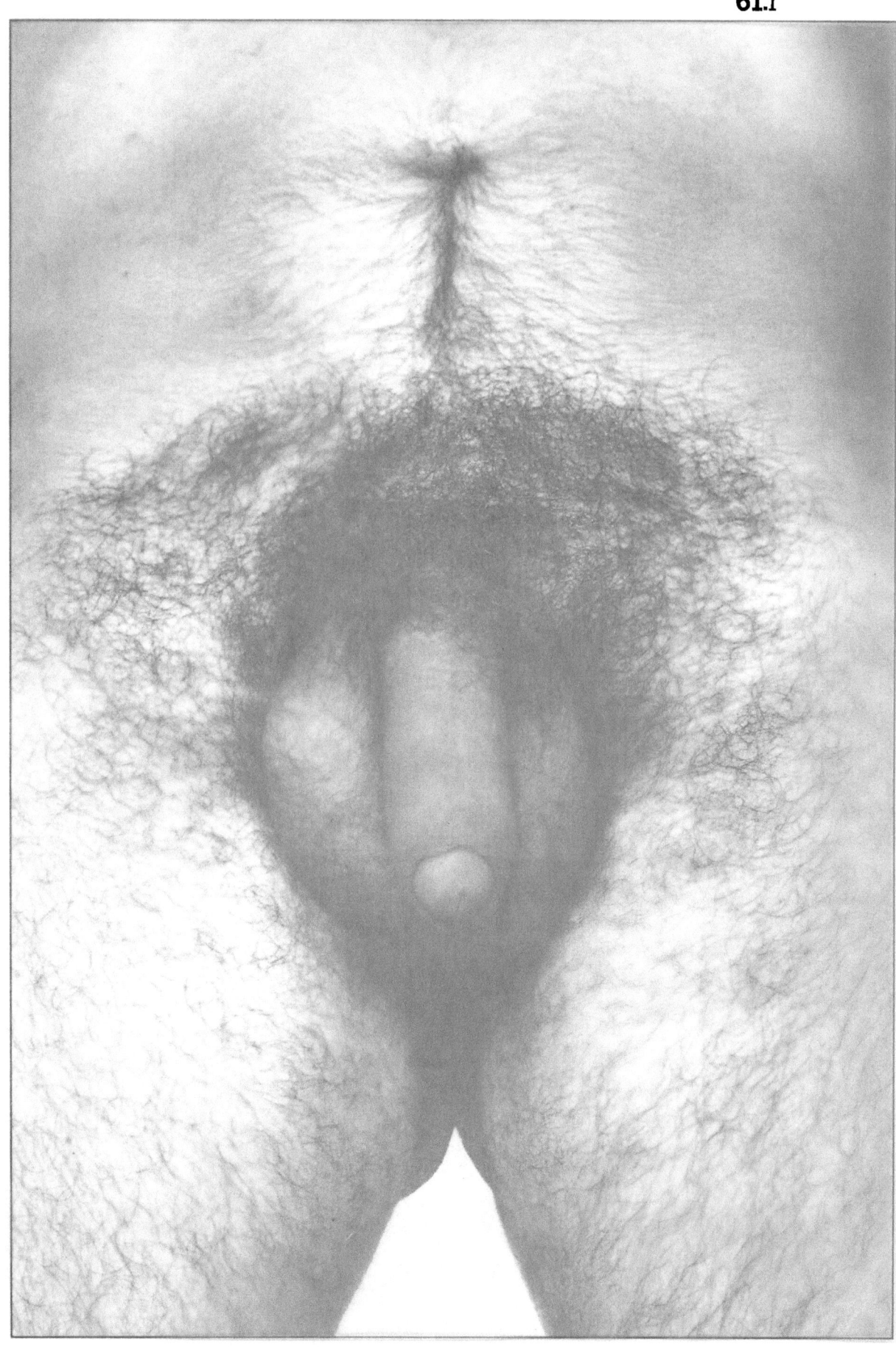

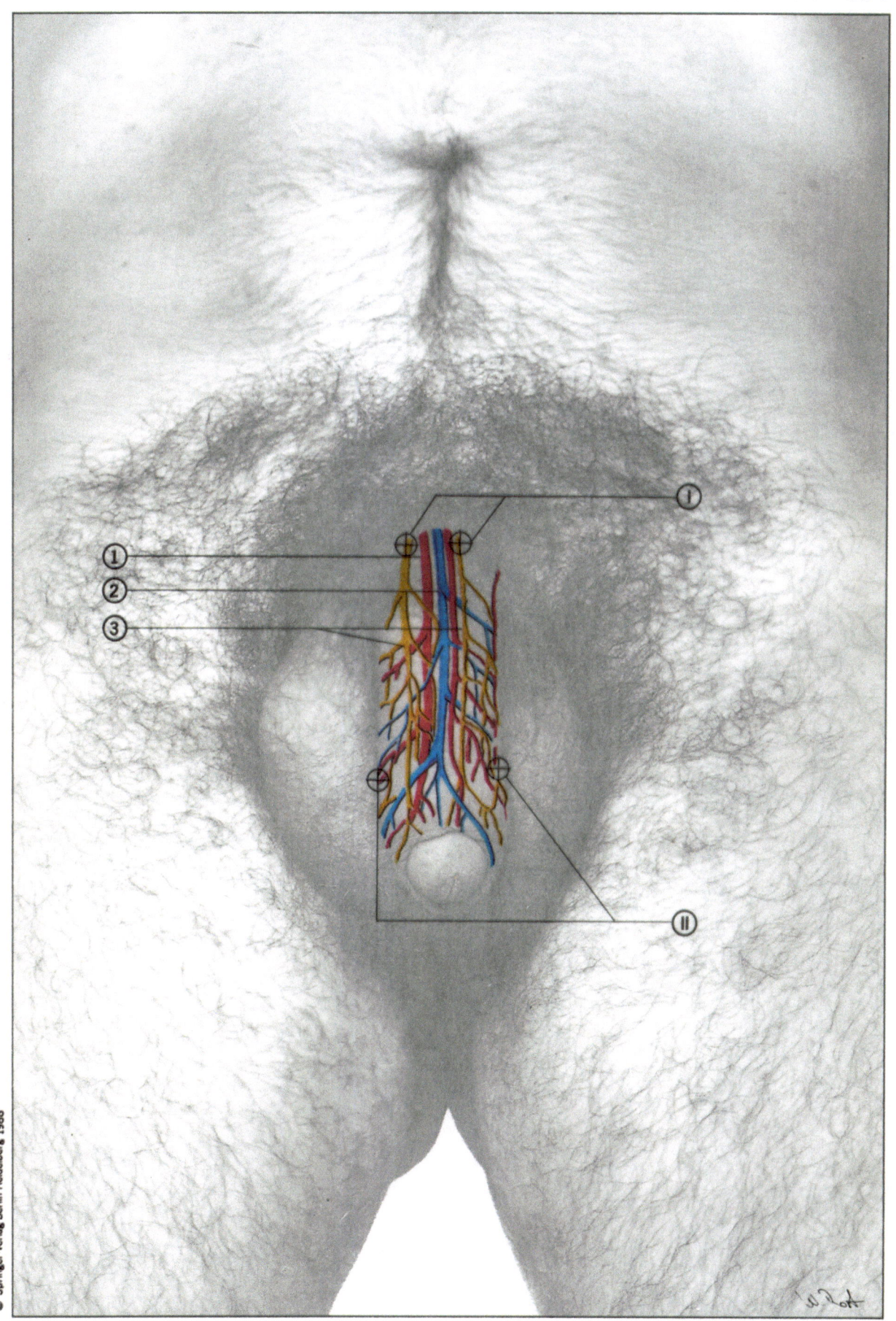

Ⓘ Points of entry for block at root of penis. ⒾⒾ Points of entry for block of prepuce. ① Dorsal penile artery. ② Dorsal penile vein. ③ Main nerve supply to penis

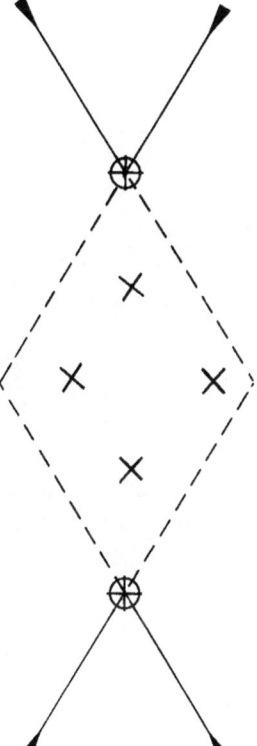

⊕ Points of entry for anal field block. ✕ Injection sites for infiltration of sphincter ani internus muscle

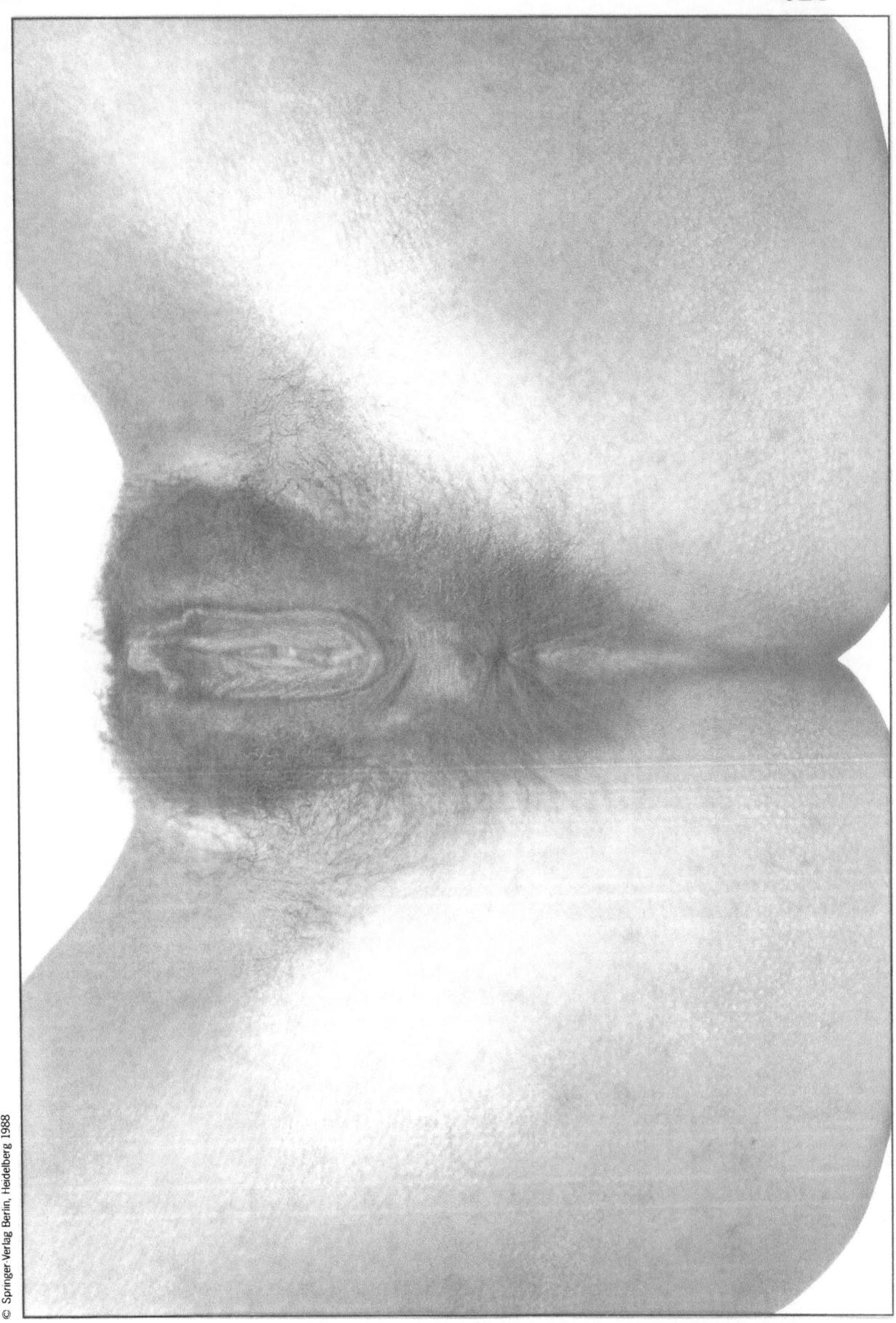

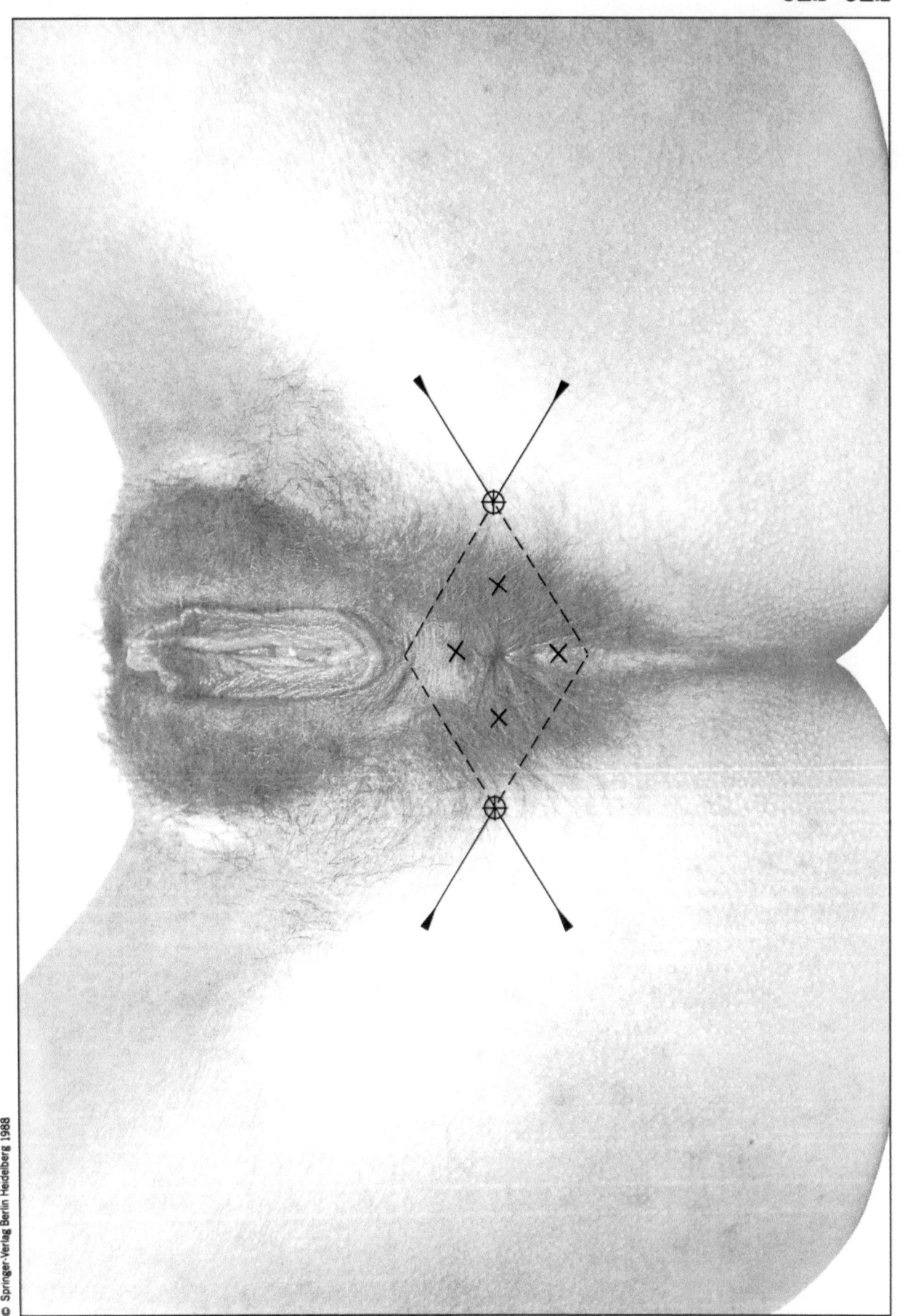

⊕ Points of entry for anal field block. ✕ Injection sites for infiltration of sphincter ani internus muscle